Lessons for MomPositive Living
Attainable Wellness for Modern Moms

Copyright © 2015 by Tammi Hoerner

The content of this book is for general instruction only. Each person's physical, emotional, and spiritual condition is unique. The instruction in this book is not intended to replace or interrupt the reader's relationship with a physician or other professional.

Please consult your doctor for matters pertaining to your specific health and diet.

The author's reference to various brands does not equal endorsement or sponsorship.

Edited by Jessica Harmon
Foreward by Lynne Dorner

To contact the publisher, visit
www.thenourishedlife.net

To contact the author, visit
www.headpositivemom.com

www.thenourishedlife.net

ISBN: 978-0-692-49040-2

Printed in the United States of America

Contents

Dedication 5

Acknowledgements 6

Foreword 7

Where it begins..9

Put it to work for you 12

Part I – MomPositive Lifestyle Habits 13

   Choose a Destination.. 14

   Journal... 16

   Breathe 32

   Improve Your Air 48

   Hydrate 64

   Speak Kindly 80

   Listen 96

   Move 112

   Sleep.. 128

Part II - MomPositive Food Habits 130

K.I.S.S. (Keep It Simple Silly!) 131

   Eat Vegetables First 162

   Eat Fruits Alone 178

   Eat Whole Grains 194

   Eat Seeds 210

   Eat Local 226

   Eat Wisely 242

   Eat Prebiotics & Probiotics.. 258

   Eat Colorfully 274

Part III – MomPositive Apothecary 290

   My Favorite Herbs & Oils 291

   Application and use of Herbs and Oils 291

   An Apothecary to Call Your Own 293

   Oil Blends & Herb recipes to experiment with.. 293

Part IV – MomPositive Recipes 295

   Coco-Yogurt Parfait 295

Peach Smoothie 295

Strawberry Bang Smoothie 296

Cran-Apple Smoothie 296

Green Smoothie 296

Happy Tummy Oats 296

Amazing Eggs and Mushroom Sauté 297

Apple Slices w/ Nut Butter 297

Strawberry Avocado Salad 297

Simple Vinaigrette 298

Rainbow of Flavor Sauté 298

Veggie Taco Chili 298

Sweet Potato Soft Tacos 298

Pizza Night 299

Broccoli Salad 299

Tri-Color Peppers & Steak 299

Burritos 299

Super Easy Grilled Chicken & Veggies 300

Putting It All Together 301

About the Author 302

MomPositive Health Coaching Resources 303

Resources & References 304

Dedication

To Jim, my forever love,
You are my rock.
To Dominik, my warrior,
You are my perseverance.
To Auriel, my lioness,
You are my creativity.
To my Granddaughter
Ava, my owl,
You are my hope.

Without each of you,
I could not be.

Acknowledgements

∞   There are so many who have played a role in the creation of this book, in both direct and indirect ways, I could not have done this without you!

∞   Mom and Dad; thank you. For loving me anyway, for pushing me to be better, for always opening your door, for rescuing me in the middle of the night, for hearing me out, and for being you.

∞   I am especially grateful to Joshua Rosenthal and the many staff at The Institute for Integrative Nutrition® who continuously pave the way for people who are passionate about being the change they want to see in this world. Thank you for giving us, your students, the support to listen to the calling we are here to fulfill, and for giving us every single tool we need to make it happen. I am eternally grateful.

∞   I am grateful to the Arenzamendi family; who all continuously teach me and my family about commitment, hard work, perseverance, focus, and solidarity, through our friendship and Taekwondo. Thank you.

∞   I am grateful to each and every one of my incredible clients who, over the years, have shared their life journey with me; every day you teach me to be a better person, a better Health Coach, and to see the world through different eyes. Thank you.

∞   To those who have inspired me to be a greater version of me along my own life journey; Erin, Sandy, Lori, and Lisa – thank you for hearing me, for guiding me, for lifting me up, for reminding me of the love in this world, and for being a bestie. You've made my journey sweeter.

∞   There are so many, many, more. You know who you are…. Thank you!

Foreword

Ever since I was a little girl, sitting on the floor playing Barbie's for days on end, I dreamed of the day I would become the *perfect* mother. All that practice! Changing their clothes, giving them baths and sitting around engaging in pretend conversations in all the different rooms of my gigantic Barbie doll house. Surely, I had role-played my way into knowing how to be a mom with ease! My family had a nickname for me-- Midget Mom because even as a 5-year-old, I was very good at organizing and dictating my family's activities. Ha! Of course, I was the youngest. The youngest of four children in a characteristically German/Irish American household. How else would I have gotten away with this queen-of-the-house behavior?

When that wonderful day arrived for me to become a real mother, Master Lexington immediately tossed me off my throne by arriving seven weeks early. I hadn't even had my baby shower yet! I knew at that moment that motherhood wasn't going to go as planned. I went into my hyper-organizing mode. The truth is that even if everything had gone as planned and my son arrived right on his due date; skipping the four days of labor; and I had had my baby shower: I still could have used some support from a seasoned mom.

In my practice as an Electrologist and a Health Coach, I have the privilege of working with moms all day long. I learn about their struggles, passions, relationships and goals. I am always striving to listen and when appropriate push my clients to reach their full potential, along the path of least resistance, in all areas of their lives. Let's face it, mothers need tools, support and sure-fire shortcuts to be modern day super moms.

My own advice has changed a lot over the years. Who wants to take advice from someone who has consistently had his or her life together and never struggled? Or from someone who isn't even a mom? I thought that the fact that I was an education major in college, a babysitter and nanny gave me permission to give moms advice. Ha! I have learned a great deal since then.

As a mom, I am now *living the dream* of constant planning, scheduling of babysitters, rescheduling them, organizing each room of our home, working around special diets, after-school programs, homework, play dates, birthday parties, haircuts, shopping, dinner preparation, bath time, bed time--and yes, that's not all! How do we do it? How do we stay positive? Is there a way to do all this with grace and love? Yes!

For the past several years I have been following Tammi Hoerner's MomPositive posts on Facebook. Always positive, eager and hopeful, I was drawn to her cheerful lifestyle. I really love her healthy recipes and inspirational posts.

Thanks to Tammi, *this* mom is now MomPositive. I am enjoying getting to know Tammi better as a colleague and a friend.

While reading Tammi's book, _Lessons in MomPositive Living: Attainable Wellness for Modern Moms,_ I was repeatedly amazed that we have so much in common. I think you too will find it easy to connect and relate with her through your own experiences with life and motherhood.

I know you will identify with many of our shared personal situations. Tammi and I were surprised to discover we're the same age! We have sons the same age. We have both been married, been single mothers and shared important healthy adult relationships. We both worked in crazy, stressful corporate jobs before starting our own businesses. We both made tough decisions about closing some businesses too! We both enjoy arranging our schedules to put our families first. We even share previous health conditions, struggles with anxiety and panic attacks, our chosen lifestyle changes have been closely aligned. We are both very sensitive and special women. Does this describe you too? If you need help to get your life in order and some inspiration from a woman who "has been through it all" and "has come out of it gracefully" this workbook is for you. Tammi isn't bitter about her life challenges ...she is better.

As mothers we all thrive on connections, short cuts, relating with one another about work, cooking in the kitchen, making better choices and working to perfect our schedules. Tammi has brilliantly put this all together in a workbook that will gently guide you, as you too 'get it all together'. Her inspiring stories, journal pages and easy recipes are ready for you to make your own. It is as if Tammi is by your side cheering you on, in your own journey to health and happiness. Enjoy your journey. Allow yourself to be the best woman and mother you can be.

Tammi's educational journey encompasses natural health, nutrition, cooking and fitness. She operates within a lovely spiritual space that is calm, peaceful and enviable. Lucky for us, she is willing to lead by example, allowing others to get out of the chaos, drama and the frenetic busyness that you will enjoy leaving behind.

As one of the first people to read *her Lessons in MomPositive Living: Attainable Wellness for Modern Moms* workbook, my first thought was: "I wish I had this the last eight years of my life." You are fortunate to have it now.

Love yourself, love your life, your schedule, your children, your work, your food, fitness and fun. Fill out out each page of this workbook and enjoy every day as you fulfill your goals and dreams.

Lynne Dorner, New York, New York
Founder and program director of *Clean Eating Programs*, author of *101+ Secrets from Nutrition School | That you Need to Know*, and contributor at *Huffington Post.* www.CleanEatingPrograms.com

Where it begins

My first and most important roles in this life are being a Mom and a Wife. My family is my strength, and everything I love in this life. Being well is vital for me to be the best Mom and Wife I can be for my family. I *must* be strong, well, focused, and balanced, so that I can teach, support, and love the way that I feel my loved ones deserve, (*As well as in the way I deserve*). Being my best self allows me the space and energy to homeschool my son and support his athletic dreams, to support and guide my daughter as she begins her own journey into motherhood, and to be a deep well of love for my incredible hard working and loving husband.

In the beginning of my own healing journey, I expected my recovery to be impossibly quick. Maybe some sort of spontaneous miracle would sprinkle down from God and miraculously change my health and life forever. I wanted this miracle to happen so I would quickly be able to return to my self-indulgent sabotaging food rituals of eating out too often, and eating foods that were toxic to me and my family when we ate in.

There are reasons for every choice we make.

Before I began my own healing journey, I found safety, quietness, and fulfillment in food. I found connection, comfort, and tranquility in food. There were things I was desperately seeking in my life that were reflected in my relationship with food. I ate when I felt sad, happy, stressed, overwhelmed, and bored. I ate when I was tired. I ate when I was celebrating. I became addicted to sugar and salt and was in a constant swing between to the two.

Then, I became ill. I never associated how I felt with the food I ate. As the pain and discomfort grew, I would try to smother it with more food.

In time, I gained weight, and I developed IBS (Irritable Bowel Syndrome), high blood pressure, high cholesterol, chronic migraines, and early onset arthritis. I was even having chest pains. *I ached all the time*. I was deeply depressed and felt horribly alone and out of control. I never realized I had a choice. I never realized that every single day, I made choices that contributed to my illnesses.

My perspective and understanding began to shift the year my eldest graduated high school and began to grow wings of her own. I was full of advice, direction, and support, hoping she'd step into the life she deserved without making all the mistakes I had. (I have made plenty of them.) I would say things like, "Don't be afraid to stand up for what you believe in," and "Find a career that resonates with and reflects *you*," and "Remember that you are in charge of what happens in your life and you can make it whatever you want to make it." As the words would tumble out of my mouth, I would hear them. I would think to myself, "*I'm not doing any of these things. Why should she follow my advice?*" What I realized in those moments was that something needed to change.

Sometimes pain is the biggest motivator and I was in a lot of it. Emotionally and physically the pain was swallowing me whole.

It was a slow uncovering of the realization that my choices in life had put me where I was, and I had to make choices to get out of it. I began to search for a solution for what was causing me the greatest pain in my life at the time – **my job**. I spent weeks pondering my interests and skills, wondering what I could do. I began to look for education that would take me in a new direction.

I found The Institute for Integrative Nutrition®. This is where my life took an incredible turn onto a beautiful path of self-healing and discovery. This path led to the carving of my new career, and a new stronger, healthier and happier version of myself.

Health: true sustainable lasting health; requires patience and commitment. On this journey there is no end; no final destination point where you get off the bus and let everything go back to the way it was. No. To lead a life bursting with energy, focus, health, and balance, you must be diligent, focused, and committed to take each day as it comes and give it all you've got. **The payoff is priceless.** By focusing on your wellbeing, you can live a life filled with happiness, light, and have the energy to follow your dreams. You become an inspiration for your family to follow suit. You become the greatest role model by leading the way.

From here on, everything will be different. Even if you choose to not use the tools you learn in this workbook, you can never un-know them. They will be there in your mind and though you may choose to look the other way at any time, you will always know the tools you learn in this book.

And so, you too have a choice.

The name MomPositive was devised by my daughter, Auriel. In a conversation we had, she shared how she had been thinking about all a mom is expected to do. The societal demands on moms today are atrocious. We are expected, by others **and ourselves** to work in a career that is financially rewarding, bear and rear healthy, happy children, keep house, garden, stay up with the latest trends, stay thin, be active, tote our children around to a million school events, cook, and maintain friendships and a healthy relationship with our hubbies. How can anyone do it all? My daughter said in thinking about it, "Well, that's not Mom-Positive." Hence, we came up with the name. I hope you'll take out the time for a Mom-Pause and step into a world where *your* **health and happiness matters**. In fact, it matters so much, the rest of everything you do depends on it!

My intention with this workbook is to give you tools that support you as you learn to make healthy choices, and to help implement these changes into your life through time management techniques, motivational journaling, and workbook questions.

In the pages that follow, you will find relevant pieces of my own journey, pieces of research, resources, and lessons that help you to integrate dynamic healthful change into your own life.

While I share these ideas, there are a few things I'd like to offer that may help you as you move forward;

∞   You are a unique being with unique needs and challenges.

∞   Listen to your brilliant body, your intuition, and your heart.

∞   Follow what feels right.

∞   Make your own rules.

∞   Set a pace that works for you.

∞   You are your best healer.

∞   You know what is right for you.

∞   The words I share here are from my experience, my journey, and what I've learned as I've worked with hundreds of women in my practice as a Certified Integrative Nutrition Health Coach.

∞   This is just the beginning of your MomPositive Life. Embrace it, call it yours, tweak it to fit your needs, and enjoy the journey!

Want more? I want to share more with you! Be sure you stop by my website to download free guides, get free recipes, and learn more from me! www.headpositivemom.com OR www.thenourishedlife.net. I am here to help you succeed!

Wishing you heaps of health, happiness, and love!

Head Positive Mom,

Jammie

Put it to work for you

This book is meant to act as an invitation to experience and think for yourself. It is also meant to act as a guide to help you implement new tools and ideas that help you to uncover your happiest, healthiest, most vibrant self!

There are hundreds, maybe thousands, of dietary and lifestyle theories in publication today. No one is perfect for everybody or every life. In this book, I invite you to think about a variety of topics, and **challenge** you to experiment with many. I give you the reflection in my life, ideas, research, and information to try in yours.

Each topic I introduce is followed by a series of questions. I hope you'll use the space provided (If you've purchased an electronic version, simply use your own paper and calendar), to write your answers and work through honestly and authentically, the thoughts to open the gateway to your inner answers.

Each series of questions is then followed by a challenge to put the topic to work for you in your life. This involves journaling and scheduling. I have included journal pages with prompts that I hope invite you to slow down and spend time with your experiences every day. By tracking your choices and thoughts around the work in this workbook, you will develop a greater understanding of what is working and why. Every topic section includes journal pages to allow you a full two weeks to practice the ideas and tools presented.

Included with every set of journal pages are scheduling areas. In these areas you might write your plans, appointments, and existing schedules – then insert the new ideas and challenges. **This process will help you practice the number one reason people do not take action – lack of time management and prioritizing.** You will learn to integrate your new habits into your already very busy schedule. By looking at what you already have planned and fitting your new lifestyle habits *around* your existing plans regularly, you'll develop a lifestyle and routine that works for you, making it **sustainable** and lifelong.

While there aren't hard steadfast rules to this, I'm hoping you'll consider using all of these pieces together.

The steps in a nutshell are:

1. Read and learn.
2. Dig deep for how this is both relevant for you and what it looks like in your life today.
3. Experiment and write into the journal pages how the new habit feels and what you notice.
4. Tuck this new action step around and through your days, developing skills and habits that are sustainable and lasting.
5. Celebrate your success!

Are you ready? Momma, YOU GOT THIS!

Part I – MomPositive Lifestyle Habits

"In the past six months, I have: gotten divorced, bought my own condo, began dating, gotten more involved in my business, gained a large supply of confidence, and experienced more freedom and happiness than I ever thought possible... I told Tammi in the beginning that fear controlled my life, now, I may feel fear but I do the things I want to do anyway! I feel like I am living an authentic life for the first time ever." – Sally Gabriel, PhD

Choose a Destination

Of all the skills I learned on this journey, one of the most valuable was the process of setting goals and developing a course of action. As children, we are always projecting into the future - dreaming of what life will be like someday - but for me in my memory, in school and at home, we never discussed it seriously until I was a young adult. Instead, I was taught to do with what I had.

There was an immense gift of resourcefulness in this which I can see clearly today. Though I kept a glass ceiling called, "I cannot afford it," and a brick wall called, "I am not good enough," around me that held me very still in personal growth and opportunity, I stopped dreaming of the future early in my "tweens", and did not pick it back up again until I met my husband.

As he and I worked to build the life we have today, we talked a lot about what our future would look like. I began to dream again of, "what life will be like when….," yet I lacked the understanding of the road map. I always felt like things came together magically, just because of what was meant to be.

As a student at IIN®, I was pulled back to my goals and vision for my life constantly. This focus became the compass and helped me to lay out the pavestones as I navigated my way through life altering information to build a career that plays a role in a much bigger picture. It's become a part of my daily practice. Every day I ask myself, "What will I create today?"

It starts with you.

In your health and life, where are you now? What about where you are do you want to change? Why do you want to change it? What will your life look like once you are in that *new and better* version of circumstances? What will open up for you? What would you reach for if you could not fail? What would you reach for if money wasn't an issue? What role does being healthy play in the bigger vision you have for your life?

Next is a simple but incredibly powerful, question: **what will it take to get there**? Can you ask this of yourself without judging or fearing the response? Are you willing to do what it will take?

Goal setting can help you break through overwhelm and create tasks that are both bite sized and realistic. Goal setting can look like many things. You can make a detailed list, a dream board, or draw pictures. You can be articulate or creative, or both!

After spending some time with the questions above, take some time to write about what you'd like to create in your life. Allow yourself the time and space to be open & honest, and to hold this space as if you were holding it for your best friend. Try not to judge as you notice what comes from your mind and heart.

After using the following journal prompts to help you get clear on what you'd like to create, refine your vision. How many things can you identify about this future you want to put together? What does it look like? What does it feel like? How old will you be? How old will your children be? How old will your partner be? What will happen once you accomplish this? Finally, wrap it with a time reference. When in your life would you like to have accomplished this by?

Begin here with this exercise.

What I'd like to create in my life is:

What will it take to accomplish my goals?

One, two, or three action steps I can take this week to help me move in the direction of my goals are:

P.S. Once you've taken the time to do this part, you've created your destination point and perhaps a nice road map for your healing journey.

Having this clarity now will help you as you move forward by knowing which ideas and opportunities are supporting you and which are distracting you from being where you want to be. You may also notice that by taking time to get clear on your goals, that your understanding of the importance of your health becomes clearer as well.

Journal

For as long as I can remember, I've kept a diary. In my earliest years, it was an evening ritual where I would write my thoughts and track the events from the day. I would tend to write more often when things were hard. This might have involved complaining about my parents, or crying over a boy. As I grew older, this evolved into a translation and record of the complexity of young adulthood events and emotions from drama at work to the challenges of being a young mom. Keeping a diary allowed me a safe space to work through my thoughts and emotions. It gave me a place of reflection and tracking where I had been.

When I began my healing journey, I added food to the mix. I started by calorie counting – writing both my exercise and foods down. This evolved into a focus on what I was doing for me that day, things that happened that I was grateful for, and writing about what I wanted to create in my life.

I still keep a journal, finding it a non-judgmental space to let go of what bothers me and a place to continuously create what I want in this life, in my body, relationships, and career.

--

Keeping a journal or a diary can be a powerful tool for life and health transformation. Writing down your thoughts and actions daily brings awareness to your choices, thoughts, and the events from day to day. You might notice habits, routines, rhythms, and cycles that you hadn't noticed before.

Taking time to write daily may help you to clarify your thoughts, get to know yourself better, understand choices you are making, reduce stress, and help you to solve problems more effectively.

There are many different approaches to keeping a journal. You can choose to write in the evening or in the morning. Some approaches involve writing down whatever comes to your mind, while others are focused on particular areas you are working on in your life.

Keeping a food journal helps to bring awareness to your food choices. Studies suggest that by developing a routine, this practice can improve weight loss success, but even if you are not seeking to lose weight, keeping a food journal can help you to identify what foods are supporting your health and happiness and which ones are holding you back. (Magee and Louise).

The most important key with food journaling is honesty. Be honest and clear with yourself. If you are working with an Integrative Nutrition Health Coach, a Dietician, or a Nutritionist, being honest in your journal gives them the tools to properly and fully support you.

--

Try this exercise

In a separate journal or spiral notebook, begin each day by writing the thoughts you have about the day before, your dreams, and what's on your mind when you wake. Allow about 30 minutes for this exercise every day when you wake for seven days. Try to write down whatever comes to your mind without judging it. No one need ever read what you are writing; even you never have to go back to read it if you choose not to. Just allow the thoughts to flow from your mind and heart to your pen and then to paper.

At the end of the seven days, answer these questions:

- ∞ What do you notice about this process?

- ∞ What are you noticing about where your focus seems to be as you write?

- ∞ Would you like to change your focus? To what?

- ∞ Is this a practice you'll continue?

Then try:

At the end of each day for seven days, take 30 minutes to write what happened during your day that you are grateful for and why it happened. You can also include how it makes you feel or how it impacts your life.

At the end of these seven days, answer the following;

What are you noticing about your life as you write these moments down?

How does this impact your life experience?

Will you keep this practice?

What are other ways you might remind yourself of the good things that happen in your everyday life?

How does this influence the way you talk to yourself?

Finally, if you haven't started yet, begin to write the foods you consume in the areas provided on the following journal pages.

You might also consider noting times you eat, why you eat, and if you want to get detailed, note calories of the foods you are consuming. An easy way to do this (thank God for technology) is to use an app. (Yes, there's an app for that!)

Here are some you can try:

myfitnesspal.com or loseit.com

If you have a Fitbit, you can use the food tracker that comes with the Fitbit application.

P.S. From this point, I've included journal pages for you to begin to track your personal journey. Using these pages will help you to track your progress, successes, and challenges. Use them to put your personal MomPositive puzzle pieces together!

DATE: _____

Morning thoughts:
_____
_____
_____
_____
_____
_____
_____

Goals & Intentions for today

1
2
3
4
5
6

6:00	
7:00	
8:00	
9:00	
10:00	
11:00	
12:00	
1:00	
2:00	
3:00	
4:00	
5:00	
6:00	
7:00	

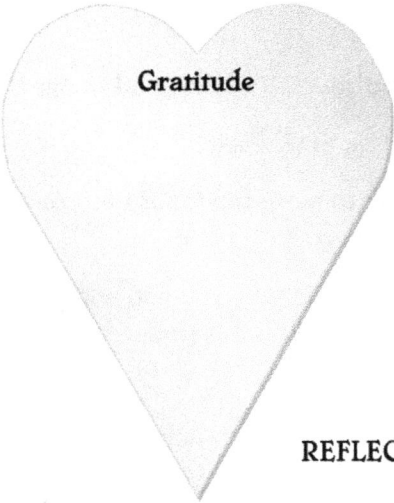

Food

Water: IIII IIII IIII

Breakfast:
_____
_____
_____

Lunch:
_____
_____
_____

Dinner:
_____
_____
_____

Snacks:
_____
_____
_____
_____

Notes:
_____
_____
_____

Gratitude

REFLECTION

_____
_____
_____
_____
_____

DATE: _____

Morning thoughts:
_____
_____
_____
_____
_____
_____
_____

Food

Water: IIII IIII IIII

Breakfast:
_____
_____
_____

Goals & Intentions for today

1	
2	
3	
4	
5	
6	

Lunch:
_____
_____
_____

Dinner:
_____
_____
_____

Snacks:
_____
_____

Notes:
_____
_____
_____
_____

6:00	
7:00	
8:00	
9:00	
10:00	
11:00	
12:00	
1:00	
2:00	
3:00	
4:00	
5:00	
6:00	
7:00	

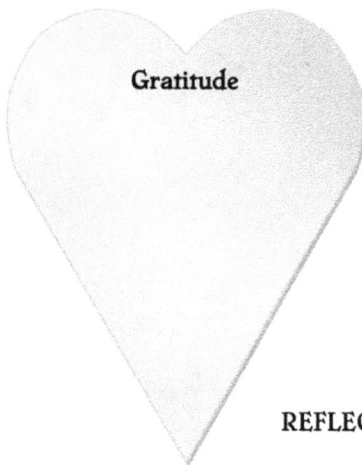

Gratitude

REFLECTION
_____
_____
_____
_____
_____
_____

DATE: _____

Morning thoughts:
_____
_____
_____
_____
_____
_____
_____
_____

Goals & Intentions for today

1	
2	
3	
4	
5	
6	

6:00	
7:00	
8:00	
9:00	
10:00	
11:00	
12:00	
1:00	
2:00	
3:00	
4:00	
5:00	
6:00	
7:00	

Food

Water: IIII IIII IIII

Breakfast:
_____
_____
_____

Lunch:
_____
_____
_____

Dinner:
_____
_____
_____

Snacks:
_____
_____
_____

Notes:
_____
_____
_____

Gratitude

REFLECTION

_____
_____
_____
_____
_____
_____

Morning thoughts:

_____
_____
_____
_____
_____
_____
_____

Food

Water: IIII IIII IIII

Breakfast:

_____
_____
_____

Goals & Intentions for today

1	
2	
3	
4	
5	
6	

Lunch:

_____
_____
_____

Dinner:

_____
_____
_____

Snacks:

_____
_____

6:00	
7:00	
8:00	
9:00	
10:00	
11:00	
12:00	
1:00	
2:00	
3:00	
4:00	
5:00	
6:00	
7:00	

Notes:

_____
_____
_____

Gratitude

REFLECTION

_____
_____
_____
_____
_____
_____

DATE: _____

Morning thoughts:
_____
_____
_____
_____
_____
_____
_____

Food

Water: IIII IIII IIII

Breakfast:
_____
_____
_____

Goals & Intentions for today

1	
2	
3	
4	
5	
6	

Lunch:
_____
_____
_____

Dinner:
_____
_____
_____

Snacks:
_____
_____

Notes:
_____
_____
_____
_____
_____

6:00	
7:00	
8:00	
9:00	
10:00	
11:00	
12:00	
1:00	
2:00	
3:00	
4:00	
5:00	
6:00	
7:00	

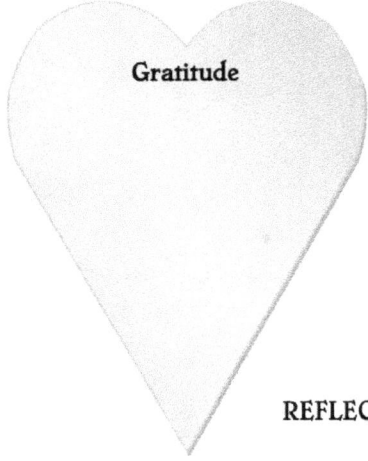

Gratitude

REFLECTION
_____
_____
_____
_____
_____
_____

DATE: _____

Morning thoughts:
_____
_____
_____
_____
_____
_____
_____

Food

Water: IIII IIII IIII

Breakfast:
_____
_____
_____

Goals & Intentions for today

1	
2	
3	
4	
5	
6	

Lunch:
_____
_____
_____

Dinner:
_____
_____
_____

Snacks:
_____
_____

Notes:
_____
_____
_____

6:00	
7:00	
8:00	
9:00	
10:00	
11:00	
12:00	
1:00	
2:00	
3:00	
4:00	
5:00	
6:00	
7:00	

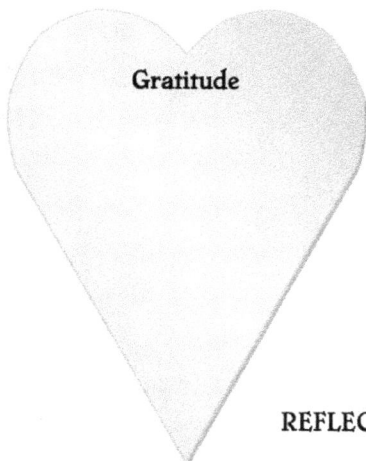

Gratitude

REFLECTION
_____
_____
_____
_____
_____
_____

23

DATE: _____

Morning thoughts:
_____
_____
_____
_____
_____
_____
_____
_____

Goals & Intentions for today

1
2
3
4
5
6

6:00	
7:00	
8:00	
9:00	
10:00	
11:00	
12:00	
1:00	
2:00	
3:00	
4:00	
5:00	
6:00	
7:00	

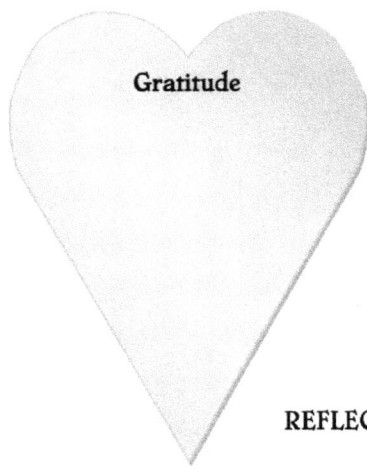

Food

Water: IIII IIII IIII

Breakfast:
_____
_____

Lunch:
_____
_____
_____

Dinner:
_____
_____
_____

Snacks:
_____
_____
_____

Notes:
_____
_____
_____

Gratitude

REFLECTION

_____
_____
_____
_____
_____
_____

24

Journal & Schedule

Morning thoughts:
_____
_____
_____
_____
_____
_____
_____
_____

Goals & Intentions for today

1
2
3
4
5
6

6:00	
7:00	
8:00	
9:00	
10:00	
11:00	
12:00	
1:00	
2:00	
3:00	
4:00	
5:00	
6:00	
7:00	

Food

Water: IIII IIII IIII

Breakfast:
_____
_____
_____

Lunch:
_____
_____
_____

Dinner:
_____
_____
_____

Snacks:
_____
_____

Notes:
_____
_____
_____

Gratitude

REFLECTION
_____
_____
_____
_____
_____
_____
_____

Journal & Schedule

Morning thoughts:

_____
_____
_____
_____
_____
_____
_____
_____

Goals & Intentions for today

1
2
3
4
5
6

6:00	
7:00	
8:00	
9:00	
10:00	
11:00	
12:00	
1:00	
2:00	
3:00	
4:00	
5:00	
6:00	
7:00	

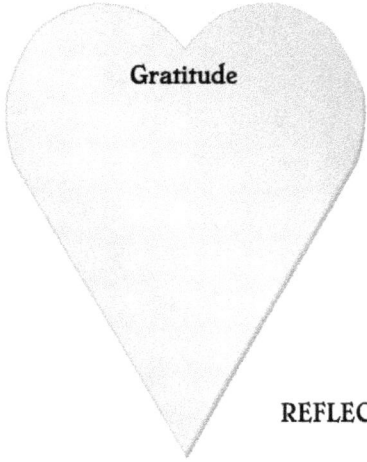

Food

Water: IIII IIII IIII

Breakfast:

_____
_____
_____

Lunch:

_____
_____
_____

Dinner:

_____
_____
_____

Snacks:

_____
_____
_____

Notes:

_____
_____
_____

Gratitude

REFLECTION

_____
_____
_____
_____
_____
_____

DATE: _____

Morning thoughts:

_____
_____
_____
_____
_____
_____
_____

Goals & Intentions for today

1
2
3
4
5
6

6:00	
7:00	
8:00	
9:00	
10:00	
11:00	
12:00	
1:00	
2:00	
3:00	
4:00	
5:00	
6:00	
7:00	

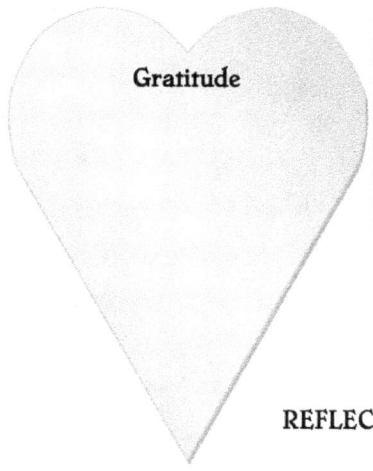

Food

Water: IIII IIII IIII

Breakfast:
_____
_____
_____

Lunch:
_____
_____
_____

Dinner:
_____
_____
_____

Snacks:
_____
_____

Notes:
_____
_____
_____

Gratitude

REFLECTION

_____
_____
_____
_____
_____
_____

Journal & Schedule

Morning thoughts:
_____
_____
_____
_____
_____
_____
_____
_____

Goals & Intentions for today

1	
2	
3	
4	
5	
6	

6:00	
7:00	
8:00	
9:00	
10:00	
11:00	
12:00	
1:00	
2:00	
3:00	
4:00	
5:00	
6:00	
7:00	

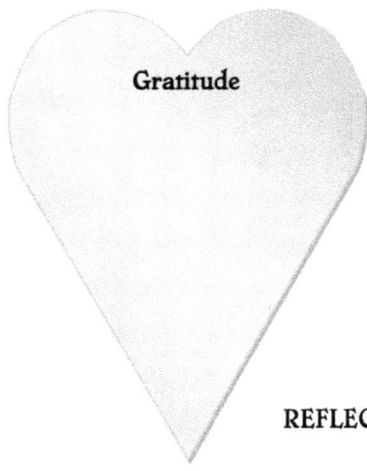

Food

Water: IIII IIII IIII

Breakfast:
_____
_____
_____

Lunch:
_____
_____
_____

Dinner:
_____
_____
_____

Snacks:
_____
_____
_____

Notes:
_____
_____
_____

Gratitude

REFLECTION
_____
_____
_____
_____
_____
_____

DATE: _____

Morning thoughts:

_____
_____
_____
_____
_____
_____
_____

Food

Water: IIII IIII IIII

Breakfast:
_____
_____
_____

Goals & Intentions for today

1

2

3

4

5

6

Lunch:
_____
_____
_____

Dinner:
_____
_____
_____

Snacks:
_____
_____

6:00	
7:00	
8:00	
9:00	
10:00	
11:00	
12:00	
1:00	
2:00	
3:00	
4:00	
5:00	
6:00	
7:00	

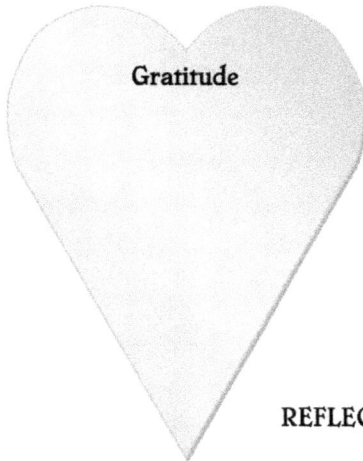

Gratitude

Notes:
_____
_____
_____

REFLECTION

_____
_____
_____
_____
_____
_____

Journal & Schedule

Morning thoughts:
_____
_____
_____
_____
_____
_____
_____

Food

Water: IIII IIII IIII

Breakfast:
_____
_____
_____

Lunch:
_____
_____
_____

Dinner:
_____
_____
_____

Snacks:
_____
_____

Notes:
_____
_____
_____

Goals & Intentions for today

1
2
3
4
5
6

Time	
6:00	
7:00	
8:00	
9:00	
10:00	
11:00	
12:00	
1:00	
2:00	
3:00	
4:00	
5:00	
6:00	
7:00	

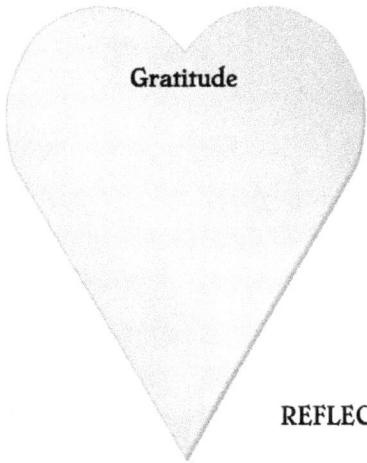

Gratitude

REFLECTION
_____
_____
_____
_____
_____
_____

Journal & Schedule

Morning thoughts:

_____
_____
_____
_____
_____
_____
_____

Goals & Intentions for today

1
2
3
4
5
6

6:00	
7:00	
8:00	
9:00	
10:00	
11:00	
12:00	
1:00	
2:00	
3:00	
4:00	
5:00	
6:00	
7:00	

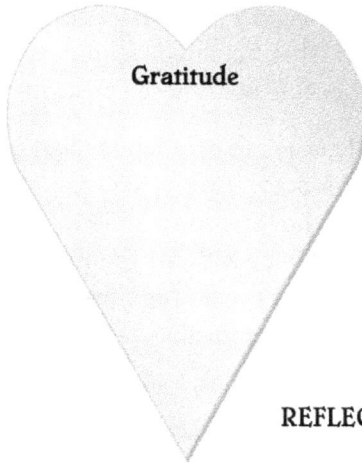

Food

Water: IIII IIII IIII

Breakfast:
_____
_____
_____

Lunch:
_____
_____
_____

Dinner:
_____
_____
_____

Snacks:
_____
_____

Notes:
_____
_____
_____

Gratitude

REFLECTION

_____
_____
_____
_____
_____
_____

Breathe

I have an enormous amount of tension in my shoulders and a sharp pain in my neck. My wrists and hands are throbbing. My eyes are heavy and I'm trying to not let on that the numbers on the screen are nothing more than a well-lit blur. I'm sure if I sit much longer, my head will take over, landing in a migraine.

I shift in my seat, glance at the clock and take my second trip to the kitchen to retrieve a pack of starburst and another cup of coffee. A small part of me acknowledges it's an excuse to move away from the poorly lit cube I spend so many hours in and work that I loathe.

My office mates are for the most part, just as miserable and display it through constant out pour of complaints and gossip. A large part of me loathes them as well. I avoid them on my way to the kitchen.

This is corporate. It is my perspective and experience. It is the ROOT of the problem in my past life.

I was doing what we do when we do with what we have and know. I was holding my breath.

In 1996, I noticed I could not seem to catch my breath. Not really short of breath like from a run, rather like the deepest inner most part of a yawn. That full opening and expansion that is so fulfilling and relaxing. That sign of enough. It started to evade me, I became ever more conscious of it. I just couldn't capture it.

It began as a light annoyance and grew into an anxiety filled experience. Days turned into weeks, weeks turned into months. I found my way to the doctor. He checked for asthma, and when seeing that even though that was ruled out, I was greatly concerned, he took some time to ask even more questions. His suggestion was to find more exercise. Move more, walk, run, play with my then very young daughter. Knowing what I know now, I can see how this would help as it would have allowed me to have a stress release. At the time, I didn't see the importance, and my commitment to adding enjoyable exercise into my busy corporate mommy life faded quickly.

It was years before this shortness of breath was under control, and even more years later before I found tools to help me completely resolve it.

I know now that many people who suffer anxiety have a tendency to hold their breath subconsciously. While anxiety is a normal reaction to stress in our life, if the stress does not let up, anxiety can become chronic and lead to a variety of stress induced reactions in the body. According to Dr. Andrew Weil, breathing exercises may be one of the single best anti-anxiety measures. (Weil)

In reflection, I was holding my breath regularly. In fact, when things get hectic, I still do. The difference is only that I am aware that I do it, and I will pause and breathe. Sometimes, I will do breath-work (just another term for breathing exercises). The difference in how I feel today is enormous and taking the time to do this prevents an all-out panic attack.

Try this exercise.

Focus on your breath. Notice and acknowledge its role in your existence. Notice how it feels to take a deep breath in; first through your nose and then through your mouth.

What do you feel as you take your breath?

What do you feel in your body as this breath comes and goes?

Learning to take time out to breathe every day can change how you feel which changes your experience, demeanor, and stress level.

Invitation to take action:

1. Sit comfortably in a chair, both feet flat on the ground. Close your eyes. Allow yourself to notice and focus on your breath. Take a long four second breath in. Hold it for five seconds, then exhale until your lungs feel empty. Try to take it to six or seven seconds. Repeat this two more times. Take time to notice how you feel before, during, and after.

2. Choose breath work to incorporate every day for seven days.

3. Is this something you'll add to your daily routine? What will you hope to achieve by the continuous practice?

Additional cool breath work techniques:

Try the breath work demonstrated by Dr. John Douillard on this youtube video:
https://www.youtube.com/watch?v=BmAZb_ShnQk

Try the breath work demonstrated by Dr. Andrew Weil on this video blog:
http://www.drweil.com/drw/u/VDR00160/Dr-Weils-Breathing-Exercises-4-7-8-Breath.html

P.S. Once I learned how valuable this was, I taught it to my son. We take three long deep breaths as we settle down to sleep in the evening. It's a little like turning down the volume and letting go of all the thoughts. Allowing and welcoming sleep to come.
P.P.S. Breathing through the mouth can produce stress signals in the brain, when you are using this method, always try to inhale through the nose to allow your body to fully relax.

Journal & Schedule

Morning thoughts:
_____
_____
_____
_____
_____
_____
_____

Goals & Intentions for today

1

2

3

4

5

6

6:00	
7:00	
8:00	
9:00	
10:00	
11:00	
12:00	
1:00	
2:00	
3:00	
4:00	
5:00	
6:00	
7:00	

Food

Water: IIII IIII IIII

Breakfast:
_____
_____
_____

Lunch:
_____
_____
_____

Dinner:
_____
_____
_____

Snacks:
_____
_____
_____

Notes:
_____
_____
_____

Gratitude

REFLECTION

_____
_____
_____
_____
_____
_____

DATE: _____

Morning thoughts:
_____
_____
_____
_____
_____
_____
_____

Goals & Intentions for today

1
2
3
4
5
6

6:00	
7:00	
8:00	
9:00	
10:00	
11:00	
12:00	
1:00	
2:00	
3:00	
4:00	
5:00	
6:00	
7:00	

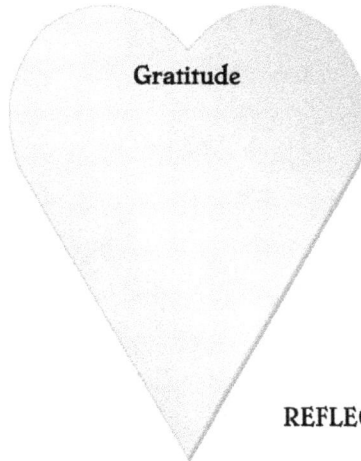

Food

Water: IIII IIII IIII

Breakfast:
_____
_____
_____

Lunch:
_____
_____
_____

Dinner:
_____
_____
_____

Snacks:
_____
_____

Notes:
_____
_____
_____
_____

Gratitude

REFLECTION

_____
_____
_____
_____
_____
_____

Journal & Schedule

Morning thoughts:
_____
_____
_____
_____
_____
_____
_____
_____

Goals & Intentions for today

1	
2	
3	
4	
5	
6	

6:00	
7:00	
8:00	
9:00	
10:00	
11:00	
12:00	
1:00	
2:00	
3:00	
4:00	
5:00	
6:00	
7:00	

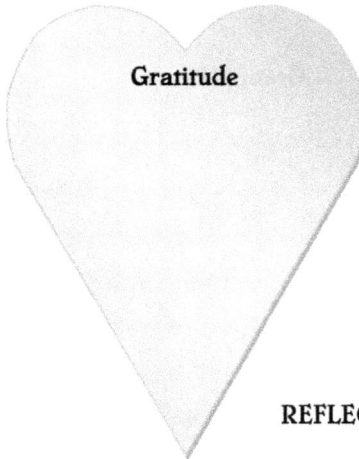

Food

Water: IIII IIII IIII

Breakfast:
_____
_____
_____

Lunch:
_____
_____
_____

Dinner:
_____
_____
_____

Snacks:
_____
_____
_____

Notes:
_____
_____
_____

Gratitude

REFLECTION
_____
_____
_____
_____
_____
_____

DATE: _____

Morning thoughts:

_____
_____
_____
_____
_____
_____
_____

Goals & Intentions for today

1
2
3
4
5
6

6:00	
7:00	
8:00	
9:00	
10:00	
11:00	
12:00	
1:00	
2:00	
3:00	
4:00	
5:00	
6:00	
7:00	

Food

Water: IIII IIII IIII

Breakfast:
_____
_____
_____

Lunch:
_____
_____
_____

Dinner:
_____
_____
_____

Snacks:
_____
_____

Notes:
_____
_____
_____

Gratitude

REFLECTION

_____
_____
_____
_____
_____
_____

DATE: _____

Morning thoughts:
_____
_____
_____
_____
_____
_____
_____

Food

Water: IIII IIII IIII

Breakfast:
_____
_____
_____

Lunch:
_____
_____
_____

Goals & Intentions for today

1
2
3
4
5
6

Dinner:
_____
_____
_____

Snacks:
_____
_____

6:00	
7:00	
8:00	
9:00	
10:00	
11:00	
12:00	
1:00	
2:00	
3:00	
4:00	
5:00	
6:00	
7:00	

Gratitude

Notes:
_____
_____

REFLECTION

_____
_____
_____
_____
_____
_____

DATE: _____

Morning thoughts:
_____
_____
_____
_____
_____
_____
_____

Goals & Intentions for today

1
2
3
4
5
6

6:00	
7:00	
8:00	
9:00	
10:00	
11:00	
12:00	
1:00	
2:00	
3:00	
4:00	
5:00	
6:00	
7:00	

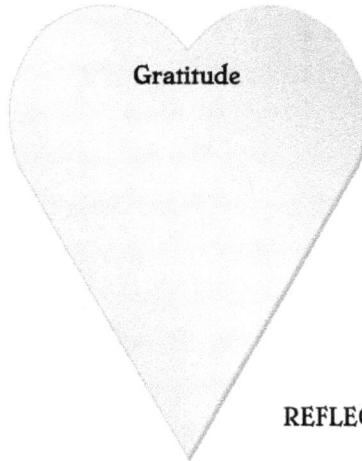

Food

Water: IIII IIII IIII

Breakfast:
_____
_____
_____

Lunch:
_____
_____
_____

Dinner:
_____
_____
_____

Snacks:
_____
_____

Notes:
_____
_____
_____

Gratitude

REFLECTION

_____
_____
_____
_____
_____
_____

DATE: _____

Journal & Schedule

Morning thoughts:
_____
_____
_____
_____
_____
_____
_____

Goals & Intentions for today

1
2
3
4
5
6

6:00	
7:00	
8:00	
9:00	
10:00	
11:00	
12:00	
1:00	
2:00	
3:00	
4:00	
5:00	
6:00	
7:00	

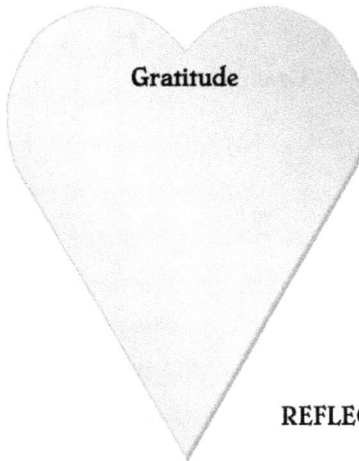

Food

Water: IIII IIII IIII

Breakfast:
_____
_____
_____

Lunch:
_____
_____
_____

Dinner:
_____
_____
_____

Snacks:
_____
_____
_____

Notes:
_____
_____
_____

Gratitude

REFLECTION
_____
_____
_____
_____
_____
_____

DATE: _____

Journal & Schedule

Morning thoughts:
_____
_____
_____
_____
_____
_____
_____

Goals & Intentions for today

1	
2	
3	
4	
5	
6	

6:00	
7:00	
8:00	
9:00	
10:00	
11:00	
12:00	
1:00	
2:00	
3:00	
4:00	
5:00	
6:00	
7:00	

Food

Water: IIII IIII IIII

Breakfast:
_____
_____

Lunch:
_____
_____
_____

Dinner:
_____
_____
_____

Snacks:
_____
_____

Notes:
_____
_____
_____
_____

Gratitude

REFLECTION

_____
_____
_____
_____
_____
_____

DATE: _____

Morning thoughts:
_____
_____
_____
_____
_____
_____
_____

Goals & Intentions for today

1
2
3
4
5
6

6:00	
7:00	
8:00	
9:00	
10:00	
11:00	
12:00	
1:00	
2:00	
3:00	
4:00	
5:00	
6:00	
7:00	

Food

Water: IIII IIII IIII

Breakfast:
_____
_____
_____

Lunch:
_____
_____
_____

Dinner:
_____
_____
_____

Snacks:
_____
_____
_____

Notes:
_____
_____
_____

Gratitude

REFLECTION

_____
_____
_____
_____
_____
_____

DATE: _____

Morning thoughts:

_____
_____
_____
_____
_____
_____
_____

Food

Water: IIII IIII IIII

Breakfast:
_____
_____
_____

Goals & Intentions for today

1	
2	
3	
4	
5	
6	

Lunch:
_____
_____
_____

Dinner:
_____
_____
_____

Snacks:
_____
_____

6:00	
7:00	
8:00	
9:00	
10:00	
11:00	
12:00	
1:00	
2:00	
3:00	
4:00	
5:00	
6:00	
7:00	

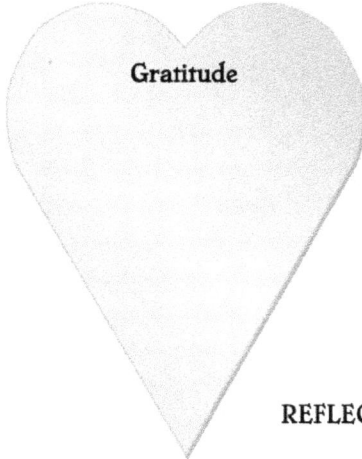

Notes:
_____
_____
_____

Gratitude

REFLECTION

_____
_____
_____
_____
_____
_____

DATE: _____

Morning thoughts:
_____
_____
_____
_____
_____
_____
_____

Goals & Intentions for today

1	
2	
3	
4	
5	
6	

6:00	
7:00	
8:00	
9:00	
10:00	
11:00	
12:00	
1:00	
2:00	
3:00	
4:00	
5:00	
6:00	
7:00	

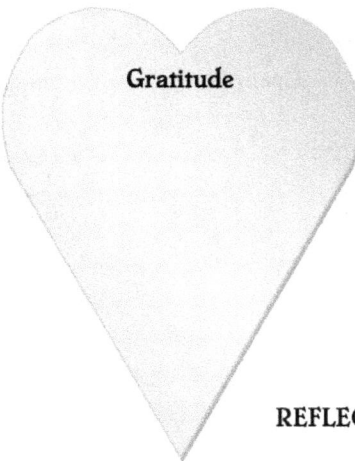

Food

Water: IIII IIII IIII

Breakfast:
_____
_____
_____

Lunch:
_____
_____
_____

Dinner:
_____
_____
_____

Snacks:
_____
_____

Notes:
_____
_____
_____

Gratitude

REFLECTION
_____
_____
_____
_____
_____
_____

DATE: _____

Morning thoughts:

_____
_____
_____
_____
_____
_____
_____

Food

Water: IIII IIII IIII

Breakfast:
_____
_____
_____

Lunch:
_____
_____
_____
_____

Dinner:
_____
_____
_____

Snacks:
_____
_____
_____

Notes:
_____
_____
_____
_____

Goals & Intentions for today

1
2
3
4
5
6

6:00	
7:00	
8:00	
9:00	
10:00	
11:00	
12:00	
1:00	
2:00	
3:00	
4:00	
5:00	
6:00	
7:00	

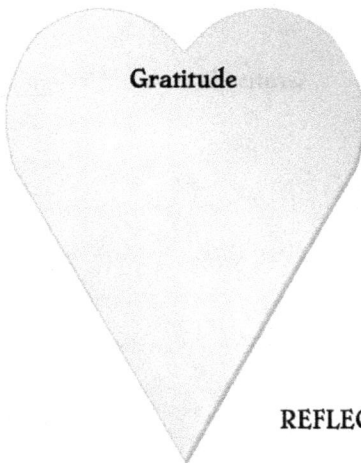

Gratitude

REFLECTION

_____
_____
_____
_____
_____
_____

Journal & Schedule

Morning thoughts:

_____
_____
_____
_____
_____
_____
_____

Goals & Intentions for today

1
2
3
4
5
6

6:00	
7:00	
8:00	
9:00	
10:00	
11:00	
12:00	
1:00	
2:00	
3:00	
4:00	
5:00	
6:00	
7:00	

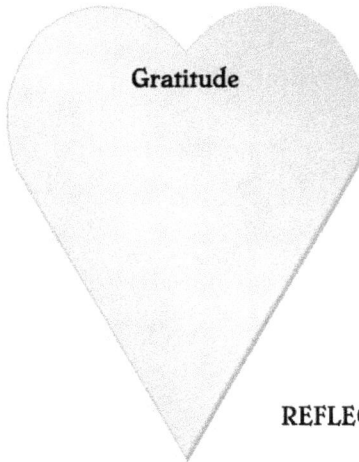

Food

Water: IIII IIII IIII

Breakfast:
_____
_____
_____

Lunch:
_____
_____
_____

Dinner:
_____
_____

Snacks:
_____
_____

Notes:
_____
_____
_____

Gratitude

REFLECTION

_____
_____
_____
_____
_____

DATE: _____

Morning thoughts:
_____
_____
_____
_____
_____
_____

Food

Water: IIII IIII IIII

Breakfast:
_____
_____
_____

Lunch:
_____
_____
_____

Dinner:
_____
_____
_____

Snacks:
_____
_____

Notes:
_____
_____
_____
_____

Goals & Intentions for today

1
2
3
4
5
6

6:00	
7:00	
8:00	
9:00	
10:00	
11:00	
12:00	
1:00	
2:00	
3:00	
4:00	
5:00	
6:00	
7:00	

Gratitude

REFLECTION
_____
_____
_____
_____
_____
_____

Improve Your Air

In the fall of 1988, a friend and I hitch-hiked to California. It was one of those late teenage rebellions I suppose – but in my mind, I was following my heart. I learned a lot on that adventure across the country, about myself and others. It's a time in my life I reference only sometimes – a time of a lot of emotional turmoil and challenge. But it's a part of my life journey none-the-less and thus a part of who I am today.

I refer to this dusty memory now as I consider times I've witnessed really poor air quality. It was in Los Angeles, my first big city visit. I don't recall noticing buildings or buses or even people. The only recollection of the city I have is that the smog was so thick and heavy, it was visible twenty five or so feet in front of me. I recall making a few comments about it, though not the words I spoke, this moment left an imprint in my memory.

Twenty some years later, the pine beetle ravaged trees in the Rocky Mountain forests caught fire. While we lived on the Eastern Plains, some distance from the mountains, the thick hot smoke hung in the air for at least two weeks after the fires were extinguished.

These are the most impactful poor air quality memories I have. I can only imagine the damage truly done by this burnt, polluted, dark air.

———

During my time at The Institute for Integrative Nutrition, our lead instructor and the founder of the school, Joshua Rosenthal gently pulled the pieces into perspective around me. He explained we can live weeks without food, days without water, but only moments without air. **A true 'A-ha' moment for me.**

Food and water clearly nourish the body, but what thought do we give to the air we breathe unless it's a labor and we are reminded of its gift? Fires and pollution from cars and factories are not all that fill our air with toxic debris. In fact, often the air we breathe indoors is more polluted than what is outdoors. Indoor air pollution is caused by recycled air, (think office or apartment buildings), carpet, furniture, and finishes such as paint that out gas toxic substances. Add toxic house cleaning chemicals to the mix and you have a recipe for disaster. How should your body respond?

This may be a part of healthy living you hadn't considered before. I know it was news for me. There are easy steps you can take to make a considerable difference in the quality of the air you breathe every day. Make these a part of your life and you'll be breathing cleaner air almost immediately.

- ∞ Change the air filters
- ∞ Keep house plants – try Aloe, Spider plants, or Golden Pothos to start – all known for their air cleaning qualities! (Knapp)
- ∞ Use an air purifier
- ∞ Open your windows
- ∞ If you have a yard, consider planting trees in it
- ∞ If you are buying a new home consider one with trees

Try This Exercise

Take a moment to answer the following to see if a few simple changes here can make a difference.

1. What do you notice about the air quality where you live?

2. How do you think this impacts your wellbeing? How about the wellbeing of your family?

3. List the top five offenders in your environment. (Do you live near a factory? A highway? In a big city?)

4. What changes can you make in order to improve the air quality in your home?

5. How does it feel to take this action?

TAKE ACTION & SCHEDULE IT!

- What will you do?

- When will you do it?

- How long will it take?

- Write it on the planner pages of this workbook. Scheduling your plan of action will make it easier to follow through.

P.S. There are a lot of ways to improve air quality and reduce exposure to toxins. I work with my clients to bring this to their awareness and take conscious action to improve one step at a time. Other areas you might learn more about include personal care products and cosmetics, house cleaning supplies, air fresheners, and even choices of fabric and materials of the products we buy. Every step in a direction to reduce, reuse, and create a healthy, natural environment is a step in the right direction.

DATE: _____

Morning thoughts:
_____
_____
_____
_____
_____
_____
_____

Food

Water: IIII IIII IIII

Breakfast:
_____
_____
_____

Goals & Intentions for today

1	
2	
3	
4	
5	
6	

Lunch:
_____
_____
_____

Dinner:
_____
_____
_____

Snacks:
_____
_____

6:00	
7:00	
8:00	
9:00	
10:00	
11:00	
12:00	
1:00	
2:00	
3:00	
4:00	
5:00	
6:00	
7:00	

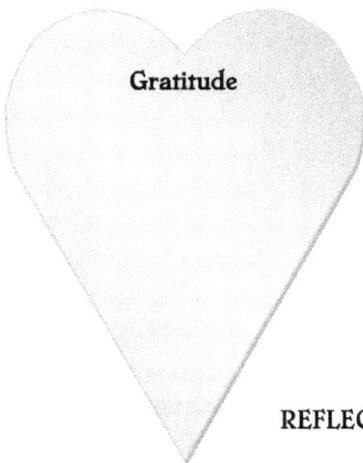

Gratitude

Notes:
_____
_____
_____

REFLECTION

_____
_____
_____
_____
_____
_____

DATE: _____

Journal & Schedule

Morning thoughts:
_____
_____
_____
_____
_____
_____
_____

Goals & Intentions for today

1	
2	
3	
4	
5	
6	

6:00	
7:00	
8:00	
9:00	
10:00	
11:00	
12:00	
1:00	
2:00	
3:00	
4:00	
5:00	
6:00	
7:00	

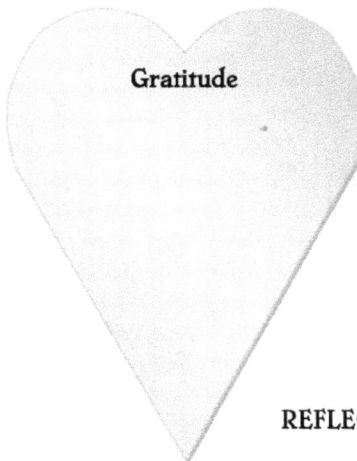

Food

Water: IIII IIII IIII

Breakfast:
_____
_____
_____

Lunch:
_____
_____
_____

Dinner:
_____
_____
_____

Snacks:
_____
_____
_____

Notes:
_____
_____
_____
_____

Gratitude

REFLECTION
_____
_____
_____
_____
_____

DATE: _____

Morning thoughts:

_____
_____
_____
_____
_____
_____
_____

Food

Water: IIII IIII IIII

Breakfast:

_____
_____
_____

Goals & Intentions for today

1	
2	
3	
4	
5	
6	

Lunch:

_____
_____
_____

Dinner:

_____
_____
_____

Snacks:

6:00	
7:00	
8:00	
9:00	
10:00	
11:00	
12:00	
1:00	
2:00	
3:00	
4:00	
5:00	
6:00	
7:00	

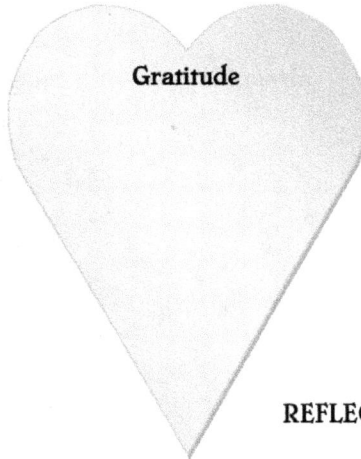

Notes:

_____
_____
_____

Gratitude

REFLECTION

_____
_____
_____
_____
_____
_____

DATE: _____

Morning thoughts:
_____
_____
_____
_____
_____
_____
_____

Goals & Intentions for today

1
2
3
4
5
6

6:00	
7:00	
8:00	
9:00	
10:00	
11:00	
12:00	
1:00	
2:00	
3:00	
4:00	
5:00	
6:00	
7:00	

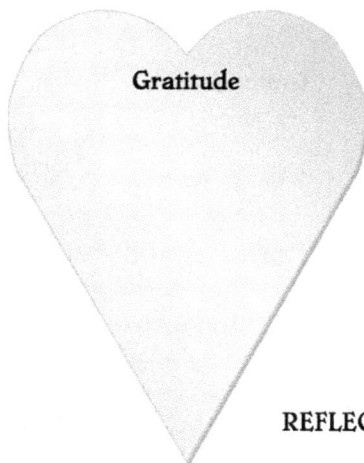

Food

Water: IIII IIII IIII

Breakfast:
_____
_____
_____

Lunch:
_____
_____
_____

Dinner:
_____
_____
_____

Snacks:
_____
_____
_____

Notes:
_____
_____
_____

Gratitude

REFLECTION
_____
_____
_____
_____
_____
_____

DATE: _____

Morning thoughts:
_____
_____
_____
_____
_____
_____
_____

Food

Water: IIII IIII IIII

Breakfast:
_____
_____
_____

Lunch:
_____
_____
_____

Goals & Intentions for today

1

2

3

4

5

6

Dinner:
_____
_____
_____

Snacks:
_____
_____
_____

Notes:
_____
_____
_____
_____

6:00	
7:00	
8:00	
9:00	
10:00	
11:00	
12:00	
1:00	
2:00	
3:00	
4:00	
5:00	
6:00	
7:00	

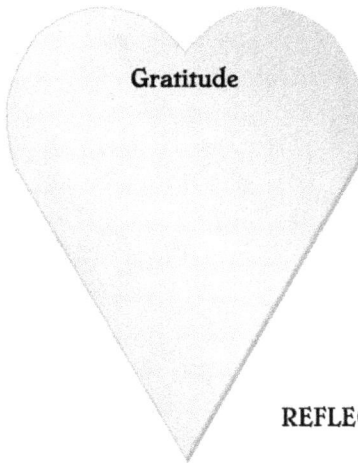

Gratitude

REFLECTION

_____
_____
_____
_____
_____
_____

54

DATE: _____

Morning thoughts:

_____
_____
_____
_____
_____
_____
_____

Goals & Intentions for today

1
2
3
4
5
6

6:00	
7:00	
8:00	
9:00	
10:00	
11:00	
12:00	
1:00	
2:00	
3:00	
4:00	
5:00	
6:00	
7:00	

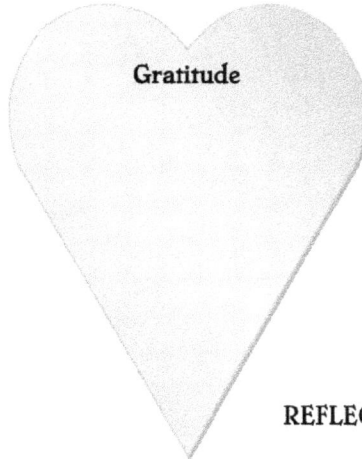

Food

Water: IIII IIII IIII

Breakfast:

_____
_____
_____

Lunch:

_____
_____
_____

Dinner:

_____
_____
_____

Snacks:

_____
_____
_____

Notes:

_____
_____
_____
_____

Gratitude

REFLECTION

_____
_____
_____
_____
_____
_____

DATE: _____

Morning thoughts:
_____
_____
_____
_____
_____
_____
_____

Goals & Intentions for today

1
2
3
4
5
6

6:00	
7:00	
8:00	
9:00	
10:00	
11:00	
12:00	
1:00	
2:00	
3:00	
4:00	
5:00	
6:00	
7:00	

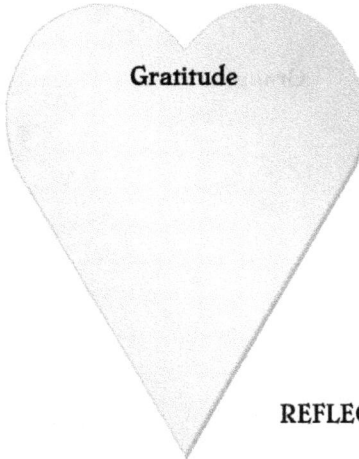

Food

Water: IIII IIII IIII

Breakfast:
_____
_____
_____

Lunch:
_____
_____
_____

Dinner:
_____
_____
_____

Snacks:
_____
_____

Notes:
_____
_____
_____

Gratitude

REFLECTION

_____
_____
_____
_____
_____
_____

56

DATE: _____

Morning thoughts:
_____
_____
_____
_____
_____
_____
_____

Food

Water: IIII IIII IIII

Breakfast:
_____
_____
_____

Goals & Intentions for today

1
2
3
4
5
6

Lunch:
_____
_____
_____

Dinner:
_____
_____
_____

Snacks:
_____
_____

6:00	
7:00	
8:00	
9:00	
10:00	
11:00	
12:00	
1:00	
2:00	
3:00	
4:00	
5:00	
6:00	
7:00	

Gratitude

Notes:
_____
_____
_____

REFLECTION

_____
_____
_____
_____
_____
_____

DATE: _____

Morning thoughts:
_____
_____
_____
_____
_____
_____
_____

Goals & Intentions for today

1
2
3
4
5
6

6:00	
7:00	
8:00	
9:00	
10:00	
11:00	
12:00	
1:00	
2:00	
3:00	
4:00	
5:00	
6:00	
7:00	

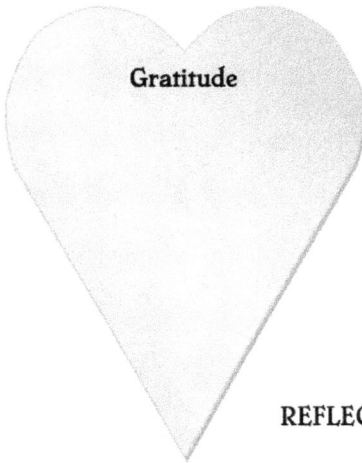

Food

Water: IIII IIII IIII

Breakfast:
_____
_____
_____

Lunch:
_____
_____
_____

Dinner:
_____
_____
_____

Snacks:
_____
_____
_____

Notes:
_____
_____
_____

Gratitude

REFLECTION
_____
_____
_____
_____
_____
_____

58

DATE: _____

Morning thoughts:
_____
_____
_____
_____
_____
_____
_____

Goals & Intentions for today

1
2
3
4
5
6

6:00	
7:00	
8:00	
9:00	
10:00	
11:00	
12:00	
1:00	
2:00	
3:00	
4:00	
5:00	
6:00	
7:00	

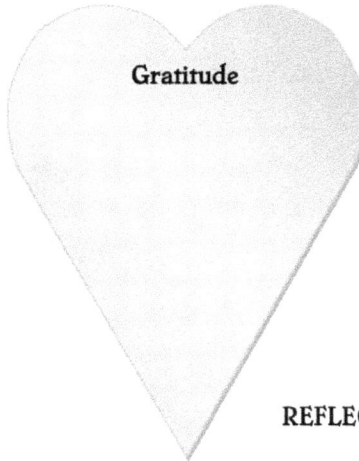

Food

Water: IIII IIII IIII

Breakfast:
_____
_____
_____

Lunch:
_____
_____
_____

Dinner:
_____
_____
_____

Snacks:
_____
_____
_____

Notes:
_____
_____
_____

Gratitude

REFLECTION

_____
_____
_____
_____
_____
_____

Journal & Schedule

Morning thoughts:
_____
_____
_____
_____
_____
_____
_____

Food

Water: IIII IIII IIII

Breakfast:
_____
_____
_____

Goals & Intentions for today

1
2
3
4
5
6

Lunch:
_____
_____
_____
_____

Dinner:
_____
_____
_____
_____

Snacks:
_____

6:00	
7:00	
8:00	
9:00	
10:00	
11:00	
12:00	
1:00	
2:00	
3:00	
4:00	
5:00	
6:00	
7:00	

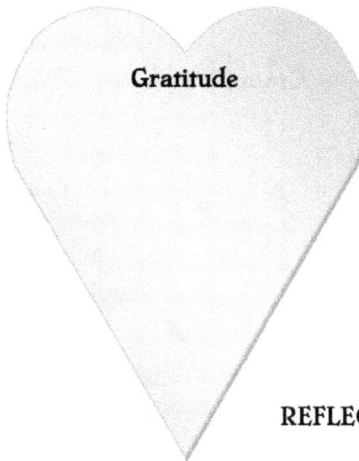

Notes:
_____
_____
_____

Gratitude

REFLECTION
_____
_____
_____
_____
_____
_____

DATE: _____

Morning thoughts:

_____
_____
_____
_____
_____
_____
_____

Food

Water: IIII IIII IIII

Breakfast:

_____
_____
_____

Goals & Intentions for today

1	
2	
3	
4	
5	
6	

Lunch:

_____
_____
_____

Dinner:

_____
_____
_____

Snacks:

_____
_____

6:00	
7:00	
8:00	
9:00	
10:00	
11:00	
12:00	
1:00	
2:00	
3:00	
4:00	
5:00	
6:00	
7:00	

Notes:

_____
_____
_____
_____

Gratitude

REFLECTION

_____
_____
_____
_____
_____

Journal & Schedule

Morning thoughts:
_____
_____
_____
_____
_____
_____

Goals & Intentions for today

1
2
3
4
5
6

6:00	
7:00	
8:00	
9:00	
10:00	
11:00	
12:00	
1:00	
2:00	
3:00	
4:00	
5:00	
6:00	
7:00	

Food

Water: IIII IIII IIII

Breakfast:
_____
_____

Lunch:
_____
_____

Dinner:
_____
_____

Snacks:
_____
_____

Notes:
_____
_____
_____

Gratitude

REFLECTION
_____
_____
_____
_____
_____
_____

DATE: _____

Morning thoughts:
_____
_____
_____
_____
_____
_____
_____

Food

Water: IIII IIII IIII

Breakfast:
_____
_____

Lunch:
_____
_____
_____

Dinner:
_____
_____

Snacks:
_____
_____

Notes:
_____
_____
_____

Goals & Intentions for today

1
2
3
4
5
6

6:00	
7:00	
8:00	
9:00	
10:00	
11:00	
12:00	
1:00	
2:00	
3:00	
4:00	
5:00	
6:00	
7:00	

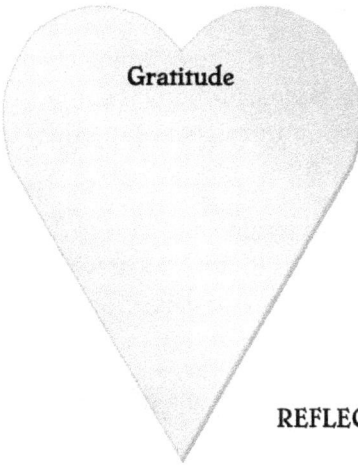

Gratitude

REFLECTION
_____
_____
_____
_____
_____
_____

Hydrate

The pain is excruciating, pulsing, blinding. If there is sound, it is amplified. If there is light, the pain is magnified.

If you've ever had a migraine, you know how it feels. I've had migraines since I was 19. I'll never forget the first, and every time I have one, I pray it will be the last. In my thirties, my incidence of migraines multiplied. I was getting them multiple times a week, for the first time, I experienced auras, and this became another layer of concern. Auras are a pulsing light in your scope of vision. Mine would become a ring and land right in front of my eyes so I could not read or write. It felt debilitating and frightening.

--

I have learned that I am far from being alone. In fact, approximately 36 million men, women, and even children suffer migraines in the United States alone (Migraine Fact Sheet). Chances are, if you've read this, you probably have had one.

It seems that there are many common factors, food triggers, and emotions that might instigate an onset of migraine headaches. From person to person this varies. If you know your triggers, you can reduce your migraine by simply making choices of foods and environments that don't set it off. **For me, dehydration is the foundation of a series of events that becomes the perfect recipe for a migraine.**

If I am well hydrated, my migraines are fewer and less severe.

What is hydration? Well, the true definition is, "to combine chemically with water." (Hydrate). This feels a little sterile but is fact even in our own living body. Our body is comprised mostly of water, which means you have water in your blood and cells. We lose water through sweat, urine, tears, and we even lose it through our skin surface.

There are many signs of dehydration, a migraine and other types of headaches are only one. You might experience dehydration through tight achy muscles or notice a craving for salty foods. You may feel light headed or have mood swings. You might even experience sleeplessness. Some experience a variety of these symptoms or even different ones.

We can fix this simply by drinking water. A good rule of thumb is to drink half your body weight in ounces of water a day. This will help you to meet the needs of your unique body. For most people, this can offer a significant change in how you feel.

Five tips for increasing water:

1. Keep it handy! Purchase a water bottle that you can have on hand always. Take it with you everywhere! (For best results, seek out a BPA Free water bottle).
2. Add fruit and herbs to it! I love adding strawberries and mint. Other blends you can try include lemon and basil, mint and cherries, cucumber and basil. Allow to steep in the refrigerator overnight.
3. Experiment with temperature. Warm, cool, hot, and cold.
4. Find an herbal tea you love.
5. Keep it simple. The less you add to the water, the easier it is for your body to use it. The more you add, the more your body has to break down before it can take the water into your cells.

Try This Exercise

For one week, drink one full glass of water upon rising. You'll want to do this before you drink any other liquids, including coffee. If you like the warmth of the coffee, try warming your water on the stove before drinking it or use a water cooler that also provides a hot water option.

Be sure to make note of your water intake in your daily journal by circling a single tab for each 8 ounce increment you consume. Do not count soda, caffeinated tea, coffee, or juice.

At the end of the first week answer the following questions.

1. How did you do?

2. What did you notice?

3. What symptoms appeared or disappeared? (Headache? Malaise? Aches? Cravings?)

4. What felt most challenging about this week's exercise?

5. How much water were you consuming each day?

6. Which day this week did you drink the most water?

7. What allowed you to succeed this day?

8. Which day did you drink the least?

9. What stood in your way?

10. Is this something you'll add to your daily diet?

11. If so, what will be your target intake daily?

12. What will you hope to achieve by including this new habit?

TAKE ACTION & SCHEDULE IT!

Continue to track your water intake daily.

DATE: _____

Morning thoughts:
_____
_____
_____
_____
_____
_____
_____

Food

Water: IIII IIII IIII

Breakfast:
_____
_____
_____

Goals & Intentions for today

1
2
3
4
5
6

Lunch:
_____
_____
_____

Dinner:
_____
_____
_____

Snacks:
_____

6:00	
7:00	
8:00	
9:00	
10:00	
11:00	
12:00	
1:00	
2:00	
3:00	
4:00	
5:00	
6:00	
7:00	

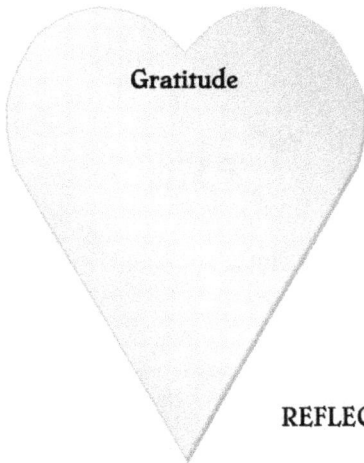

Gratitude

Notes:
_____
_____

REFLECTION

_____
_____
_____
_____
_____
_____

DATE: _____

Morning thoughts:
_____
_____
_____
_____
_____
_____
_____

Food

Water: IIII IIII IIII

Breakfast:
_____
_____
_____

Goals & Intentions for today

1
2
3
4
5
6

Lunch:
_____
_____
_____

Dinner:
_____
_____
_____

Snacks:
_____
_____

6:00	
7:00	
8:00	
9:00	
10:00	
11:00	
12:00	
1:00	
2:00	
3:00	
4:00	
5:00	
6:00	
7:00	

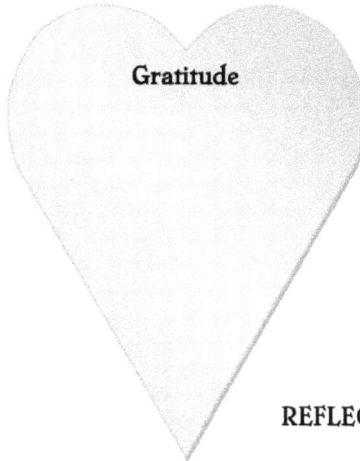

Gratitude

Notes:
_____
_____
_____

REFLECTION

_____
_____
_____
_____
_____

Journal & Schedule

Morning thoughts:
_____
_____
_____
_____
_____
_____
_____

Goals & Intentions for today

1
2
3
4
5
6

6:00	
7:00	
8:00	
9:00	
10:00	
11:00	
12:00	
1:00	
2:00	
3:00	
4:00	
5:00	
6:00	
7:00	

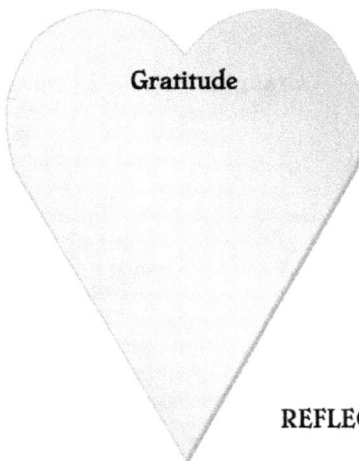

Food

Water: IIII IIII IIII

Breakfast:
_____
_____
_____

Lunch:
_____
_____
_____

Dinner:
_____
_____
_____

Snacks:
_____
_____

Notes:
_____
_____
_____

Gratitude

REFLECTION
_____
_____
_____
_____
_____
_____

DATE: _____

Morning thoughts:
_____
_____
_____
_____
_____
_____
_____

Goals & Intentions for today

1
2
3
4
5
6

6:00	
7:00	
8:00	
9:00	
10:00	
11:00	
12:00	
1:00	
2:00	
3:00	
4:00	
5:00	
6:00	
7:00	

Food

Water: IIII IIII IIII

Breakfast:
_____
_____
_____

Lunch:
_____
_____
_____

Dinner:
_____
_____
_____

Snacks:
_____
_____
_____

Notes:
_____
_____
_____
_____

Gratitude

REFLECTION
_____
_____
_____
_____
_____
_____

DATE: _____

Morning thoughts:
_____
_____
_____
_____
_____
_____
_____

Goals & Intentions for today

1
2
3
4
5
6

6:00	
7:00	
8:00	
9:00	
10:00	
11:00	
12:00	
1:00	
2:00	
3:00	
4:00	
5:00	
6:00	
7:00	

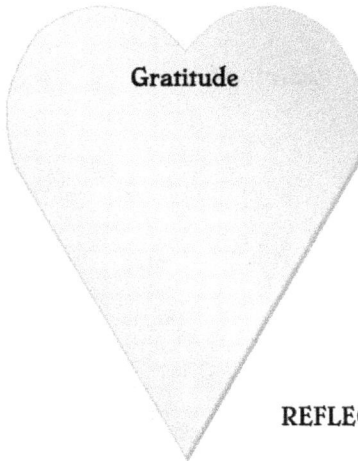

Food

Water: IIII IIII IIII

Breakfast:
_____
_____
_____

Lunch:
_____
_____
_____

Dinner:
_____
_____

Snacks:
_____
_____

Notes:
_____
_____
_____
_____

Gratitude

REFLECTION
_____
_____
_____
_____
_____
_____

DATE: _____

Morning thoughts:
_____
_____
_____
_____
_____
_____
_____

Food

Water: IIII IIII IIII

Breakfast:
_____
_____
_____

Lunch:
_____
_____
_____

Goals & Intentions for today

1	
2	
3	
4	
5	
6	

Dinner:
_____
_____
_____

Snacks:
_____
_____

6:00	
7:00	
8:00	
9:00	
10:00	
11:00	
12:00	
1:00	
2:00	
3:00	
4:00	
5:00	
6:00	
7:00	

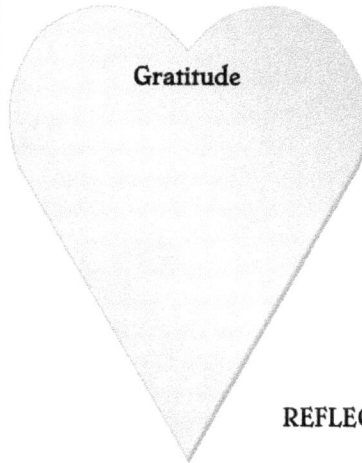

Notes:
_____
_____
_____

Gratitude

REFLECTION

_____
_____
_____
_____
_____
_____

DATE: _____

Journal & Schedule

Morning thoughts:
_____
_____
_____
_____
_____
_____
_____

Goals & Intentions for today

1
2
3
4
5
6

6:00	
7:00	
8:00	
9:00	
10:00	
11:00	
12:00	
1:00	
2:00	
3:00	
4:00	
5:00	
6:00	
7:00	

Food

Water: IIII IIII IIII

Breakfast:
_____
_____
_____

Lunch:
_____
_____
_____

Dinner:
_____
_____
_____

Snacks:
_____
_____
_____

Notes:
_____
_____
_____

Gratitude

REFLECTION
_____
_____
_____
_____
_____
_____

DATE: _____

Morning thoughts:
_____
_____
_____
_____
_____
_____

Goals & Intentions for today

1

2

3

4

5

6

6:00	
7:00	
8:00	
9:00	
10:00	
11:00	
12:00	
1:00	
2:00	
3:00	
4:00	
5:00	
6:00	
7:00	

Gratitude

REFLECTION

_____
_____
_____
_____
_____

Food

Water: IIII IIII IIII

Breakfast:
_____
_____
_____

Lunch:
_____
_____
_____

Dinner:
_____
_____
_____

Snacks:
_____
_____
_____

Notes:
_____
_____
_____

Journal & Schedule

DATE: _____

Morning thoughts:

_____
_____
_____
_____
_____
_____
_____

Goals & Intentions for today

1	
2	
3	
4	
5	
6	

6:00	
7:00	
8:00	
9:00	
10:00	
11:00	
12:00	
1:00	
2:00	
3:00	
4:00	
5:00	
6:00	
7:00	

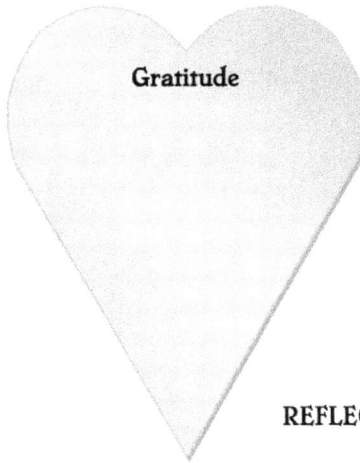

Food

Water: IIII IIII IIII

Breakfast:
_____
_____
_____

Lunch:
_____
_____
_____

Dinner:
_____
_____
_____

Snacks:
_____
_____
_____

Notes:
_____
_____
_____

Gratitude

REFLECTION

_____
_____
_____
_____
_____
_____

Journal & Schedule

Morning thoughts:
_____
_____
_____
_____
_____
_____
_____

Food

Water: IIII IIII IIII

Breakfast:
_____
_____
_____

Goals & Intentions for today

1
2
3
4
5
6

Lunch:
_____
_____
_____

Dinner:
_____
_____
_____

Snacks:
_____
_____
_____

6:00	
7:00	
8:00	
9:00	
10:00	
11:00	
12:00	
1:00	
2:00	
3:00	
4:00	
5:00	
6:00	
7:00	

Notes:
_____
_____
_____

Gratitude

REFLECTION

_____
_____
_____
_____
_____
_____

DATE: _____

Food

Water: IIII IIII IIII

Morning thoughts:
_____
_____
_____
_____
_____
_____
_____

Breakfast:
_____
_____
_____

Lunch:
_____
_____
_____

Goals & Intentions for today

1
2
3
4
5
6

Dinner:
_____
_____
_____

Snacks:
_____
_____

Notes:
_____
_____
_____
_____

6:00	
7:00	
8:00	
9:00	
10:00	
11:00	
12:00	
1:00	
2:00	
3:00	
4:00	
5:00	
6:00	
7:00	

Gratitude

REFLECTION

_____
_____
_____
_____
_____
_____

DATE: _____

Morning thoughts:
_____
_____
_____
_____
_____
_____
_____

Goals & Intentions for today

1	
2	
3	
4	
5	
6	

6:00	
7:00	
8:00	
9:00	
10:00	
11:00	
12:00	
1:00	
2:00	
3:00	
4:00	
5:00	
6:00	
7:00	

Food

Water: IIII IIII IIII

Breakfast:
_____
_____
_____

Lunch:
_____
_____
_____

Dinner:
_____
_____
_____

Snacks:
_____
_____

Notes:
_____
_____
_____

Gratitude

REFLECTION
_____
_____
_____
_____

Journal & Schedule

Morning thoughts:
_____
_____
_____
_____
_____
_____
_____

Food

Water: IIII IIII IIII

Breakfast:
_____
_____
_____

Goals & Intentions for today

1

2

3

4

5

6

Lunch:
_____
_____
_____

Dinner:
_____
_____
_____

Snacks:
_____
_____
_____

6:00	
7:00	
8:00	
9:00	
10:00	
11:00	
12:00	
1:00	
2:00	
3:00	
4:00	
5:00	
6:00	
7:00	

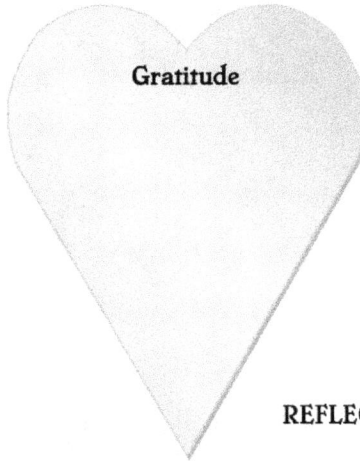

Notes:
_____
_____
_____

Gratitude

REFLECTION

_____
_____
_____
_____
_____
_____

DATE: _____

Morning thoughts:

_____
_____
_____
_____
_____
_____
_____

Food

Water: IIII IIII IIII

Breakfast:
_____
_____
_____

Lunch:
_____
_____
_____

Dinner:
_____
_____
_____

Snacks:
_____
_____
_____

Notes:
_____
_____
_____
_____

Goals & Intentions for today

1	
2	
3	
4	
5	
6	

6:00	
7:00	
8:00	
9:00	
10:00	
11:00	
12:00	
1:00	
2:00	
3:00	
4:00	
5:00	
6:00	
7:00	

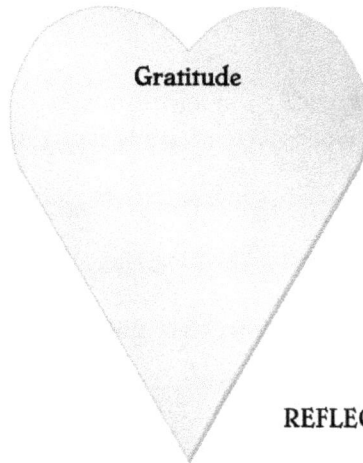

Gratitude

REFLECTION

_____
_____
_____
_____
_____
_____

Speak Kindly

"What's wrong with me?" "I did it again! I am so out of control!" "What do I matter?" "I just can't!!" "I'll never be pretty." "What's happening to me?"

In the past, these are all words and questions I repeatedly used with myself, especially when things didn't go the way I wanted. In fact, I spent the first half of my life feeling like I didn't fit in, that I wasn't in charge, that I was never going to succeed, that I was a victim.

When I learned that the language I chose in both my thoughts and conversation with others had power over the experience I was having, I made a permanent shift. My life experience, satisfaction, and opportunities unfolded like a flower.

--

What power is in a word spoken? How might you be creating your life by words you speak to yourself and to others? What experience are you creating? Do you speak kindly? Lovingly? Patiently? Are you short? Cruel? Belittling?

A brilliant scientist and author, Dr. Emoto brought an idea to the scientific table that water might actually change structure according to the energy or feelings that were directed toward it. These experiments led to a beautiful and powerful discovery. The water would change its crystalline structure according to the emotion, blessing, prayer, or intention sent to it. It's interesting to ponder; especially when you consider that our body is between 65% and 80% water.

Affirmations are words we speak and read to ourselves to help us to redefine our relationship with ourselves and the world around us. They are words we can use to gain perspective, understanding, and balance.

Suggested reading, websites, and authors;

- The Secret, by Rhonda Byrne
- Louise Hay at louisehay.com
- Sending Love to Water, Dr. Masaru Emoto: - https://youtu.be/2_dmYT83ZKY

Practice speaking kindly to yourself and others. Here are a few tips to help you:

- ∞ Use this journal to write about this idea. How are you currently speaking to yourself? How might it impact your choices throughout the day?
- ∞ Write affirmations in dry erase marker on your mirror.
- ∞ Try writing inspiring, motivating ideas and thoughts that resonate with you on a sticky note and attach them to your computer screen.
- ∞ Surround yourself with positive messages.
- ∞ Create a vision board that represents the happiness you'd like to create in your life.

Try this exercise:

Identify one or two affirmations that resonate with you. You can create these yourself or Google them! (*Isn't the internet cool?*) You are already a gifted, brilliant, being of light. Remind yourself that you deserve a life filled with vibrancy and abundant love!

An affirmation usually begins with "I Am" and should be in the present tense, specific, and positive.

Here are a few examples:

I am surrounded by love.

I am well and filled with energy every day.

I am blessed by an abundant life.

Money flows to me freely and easily.

I attract those who are meant to benefit from my work.

I treat my body well because I deserve to live a full and healthy life.

Once you've identified the affirmations which you'd like to focus on, write them down where you can refer to them frequently. The more you refer to them, repeat them to yourself, or out loud, the more benefit you will find. Try writing them in the calendar pages of this workbook.

Do this for 14 days.

At the end of 14 days, answer the following:

Have you referred to your affirmations?

What did you learn from this practice that you would like to put to work in your life?

Please write your affirmations here:

What affirmations would you like to include in the future?

P.S. Take this to the next level and consider taping loving and affirming messages to your water bottle.

P.P.S. Imagine learning this as a young child how different your experience might be. Sharing empowering and loving messages with your children can help them to make this a habit that shapes their own life experience.

DATE: _____

Morning thoughts:
_____
_____
_____
_____
_____
_____
_____

Food

Water: IIII IIII IIII

Breakfast:
_____
_____
_____

Lunch:
_____
_____
_____

Goals & Intentions for today

1	
2	
3	
4	
5	
6	

Dinner:
_____
_____
_____

Snacks:
_____
_____

Notes:
_____
_____
_____

6:00	
7:00	
8:00	
9:00	
10:00	
11:00	
12:00	
1:00	
2:00	
3:00	
4:00	
5:00	
6:00	
7:00	

Gratitude

REFLECTION

_____
_____
_____
_____
_____
_____

DATE: _____

Morning thoughts:
_____
_____
_____
_____
_____
_____
_____

Food

Water: IIII IIII IIII

Breakfast:
_____
_____
_____

Lunch:
_____
_____
_____

Dinner:
_____
_____
_____

Snacks:
_____
_____
_____

Notes:
_____
_____
_____

Goals & Intentions for today

1	
2	
3	
4	
5	
6	

6:00	
7:00	
8:00	
9:00	
10:00	
11:00	
12:00	
1:00	
2:00	
3:00	
4:00	
5:00	
6:00	
7:00	

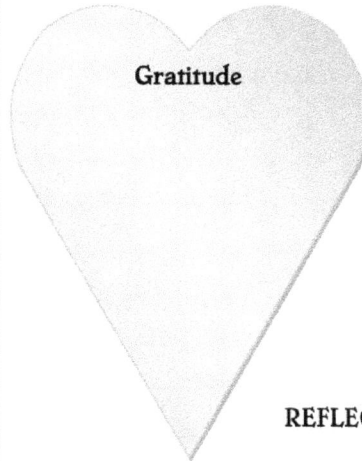

Gratitude

REFLECTION
_____
_____
_____
_____
_____

DATE: _____

Morning thoughts:
_____
_____
_____
_____
_____
_____
_____

Food

Water: IIII IIII IIII

Breakfast:
_____
_____
_____

Goals & Intentions for today

1	
2	
3	
4	
5	
6	

Lunch:
_____
_____
_____

Dinner:
_____
_____
_____

Snacks:
_____
_____

6:00	
7:00	
8:00	
9:00	
10:00	
11:00	
12:00	
1:00	
2:00	
3:00	
4:00	
5:00	
6:00	
7:00	

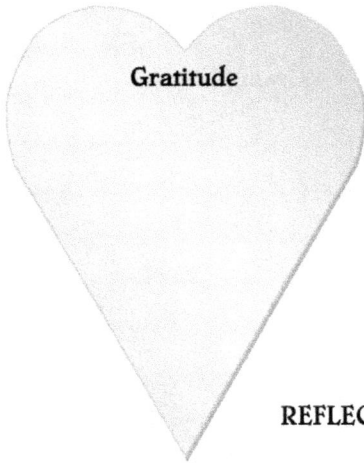

Gratitude

Notes:
_____
_____
_____

REFLECTION

_____
_____
_____
_____
_____
_____

DATE: _____

Morning thoughts:

_____
_____
_____
_____
_____
_____
_____

Food

Water: IIII IIII IIII

Breakfast:
_____
_____
_____

Goals & Intentions for today

1
2
3
4
5
6

Lunch:
_____
_____
_____

Dinner:
_____
_____
_____

Snacks:
_____

6:00	
7:00	
8:00	
9:00	
10:00	
11:00	
12:00	
1:00	
2:00	
3:00	
4:00	
5:00	
6:00	
7:00	

Notes:
_____
_____

Gratitude

REFLECTION

_____
_____
_____
_____
_____
_____

DATE: _____

Morning thoughts:
_____
_____
_____
_____
_____
_____
_____

Food

Water: IIII IIII IIII

Breakfast:
_____
_____
_____

Goals & Intentions for today

1
2
3
4
5
6

Lunch:
_____
_____
_____

Dinner:
_____
_____
_____

6:00	
7:00	
8:00	
9:00	
10:00	
11:00	
12:00	
1:00	
2:00	
3:00	
4:00	
5:00	
6:00	
7:00	

Snacks:
_____
_____

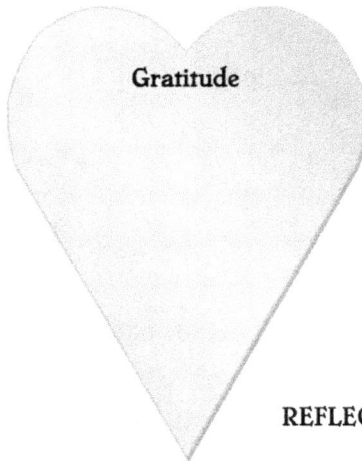

Gratitude

Notes:
_____
_____
_____

REFLECTION
_____
_____
_____
_____
_____
_____

86

Journal & Schedule

Morning thoughts:
_____
_____
_____
_____
_____
_____
_____

Goals & Intentions for today

1
2
3
4
5
6

6:00	
7:00	
8:00	
9:00	
10:00	
11:00	
12:00	
1:00	
2:00	
3:00	
4:00	
5:00	
6:00	
7:00	

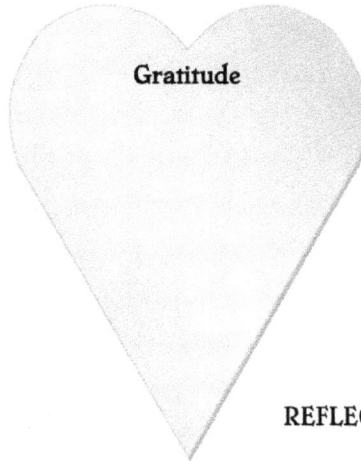

Food

Water: IIII IIII IIII

Breakfast:
_____
_____
_____

Lunch:
_____
_____
_____

Dinner:
_____
_____
_____

Snacks:
_____
_____

Notes:
_____
_____
_____

Gratitude

REFLECTION

_____
_____
_____
_____
_____

DATE: _____

Morning thoughts:
_____
_____
_____
_____
_____
_____
_____

Goals & Intentions for today

1
2
3
4
5
6

6:00	
7:00	
8:00	
9:00	
10:00	
11:00	
12:00	
1:00	
2:00	
3:00	
4:00	
5:00	
6:00	
7:00	

Gratitude

Food

Water: IIII IIII IIII

Breakfast:
_____
_____
_____

Lunch:
_____
_____
_____

Dinner:
_____
_____
_____

Snacks:
_____
_____
_____

Notes:
_____
_____
_____

REFLECTION
_____
_____
_____
_____
_____

Journal & Schedule

Morning thoughts:

_____
_____
_____
_____
_____
_____
_____

Food

Water: IIII IIII IIII

Breakfast:
_____
_____
_____

Goals & Intentions for today

1	
2	
3	
4	
5	
6	

Lunch:
_____
_____
_____

Dinner:
_____
_____
_____

Snacks:
_____
_____

6:00	
7:00	
8:00	
9:00	
10:00	
11:00	
12:00	
1:00	
2:00	
3:00	
4:00	
5:00	
6:00	
7:00	

Notes:
_____
_____
_____

Gratitude

REFLECTION

_____
_____
_____
_____
_____
_____

Journal & Schedule

Morning thoughts:
_____
_____
_____
_____
_____
_____
_____

Goals & Intentions for today

1	
2	
3	
4	
5	
6	

6:00	
7:00	
8:00	
9:00	
10:00	
11:00	
12:00	
1:00	
2:00	
3:00	
4:00	
5:00	
6:00	
7:00	

Food

Water: IIII IIII IIII

Breakfast:
_____
_____
_____

Lunch:
_____
_____
_____

Dinner:
_____
_____
_____

Snacks:
_____
_____

Notes:
_____
_____
_____

Gratitude

REFLECTION
_____
_____
_____
_____
_____
_____

DATE: _____

Morning thoughts:

_____
_____
_____
_____
_____
_____
_____

Food

Water: IIII IIII IIII

Breakfast:
_____
_____
_____

Lunch:
_____
_____
_____

Dinner:
_____
_____
_____

Snacks:
_____
_____
_____

Notes:
_____
_____
_____
_____

Goals & Intentions for today

1
2
3
4
5
6

6:00	
7:00	
8:00	
9:00	
10:00	
11:00	
12:00	
1:00	
2:00	
3:00	
4:00	
5:00	
6:00	
7:00	

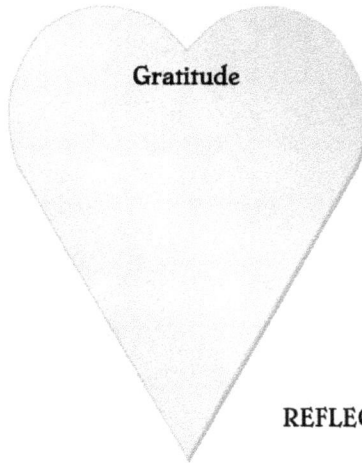

Gratitude

REFLECTION

_____
_____
_____
_____
_____
_____

DATE: _____

Morning thoughts:

_____
_____
_____
_____
_____
_____
_____

Goals & Intentions for today

1
2
3
4
5
6

6:00	
7:00	
8:00	
9:00	
10:00	
11:00	
12:00	
1:00	
2:00	
3:00	
4:00	
5:00	
6:00	
7:00	

Food

Water: IIII IIII IIII

Breakfast:
_____
_____

Lunch:
_____
_____
_____

Dinner:
_____
_____
_____

Snacks:
_____
_____
_____

Notes:
_____
_____
_____

Gratitude

REFLECTION

_____
_____
_____
_____
_____
_____

DATE: _____

Morning thoughts:
_____
_____
_____
_____
_____
_____
_____

Goals & Intentions for today

1
2
3
4
5
6

6:00	
7:00	
8:00	
9:00	
10:00	
11:00	
12:00	
1:00	
2:00	
3:00	
4:00	
5:00	
6:00	
7:00	

Food

Water: IIII IIII IIII

Breakfast:
_____
_____
_____

Lunch:
_____
_____
_____

Dinner:
_____
_____
_____

Snacks:
_____
_____

Notes:
_____
_____
_____

Gratitude

REFLECTION
_____
_____
_____
_____
_____
_____

DATE: _____

Morning thoughts:
_____
_____
_____
_____
_____
_____
_____

Food

Water: IIII IIII IIII

Breakfast:
_____
_____

Lunch:
_____
_____
_____

Dinner:
_____
_____

Snacks:
_____
_____

Notes:
_____
_____
_____

Goals & Intentions for today

1
2
3
4
5
6

Time	
6:00	
7:00	
8:00	
9:00	
10:00	
11:00	
12:00	
1:00	
2:00	
3:00	
4:00	
5:00	
6:00	
7:00	

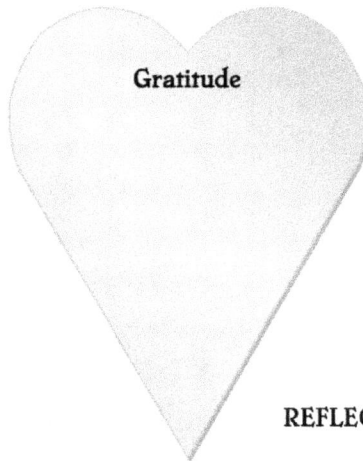

Gratitude

REFLECTION
_____
_____
_____
_____
_____
_____

DATE: _____

Morning thoughts:

_____
_____
_____
_____
_____
_____
_____

Goals & Intentions for today

1
2
3
4
5
6

6:00	
7:00	
8:00	
9:00	
10:00	
11:00	
12:00	
1:00	
2:00	
3:00	
4:00	
5:00	
6:00	
7:00	

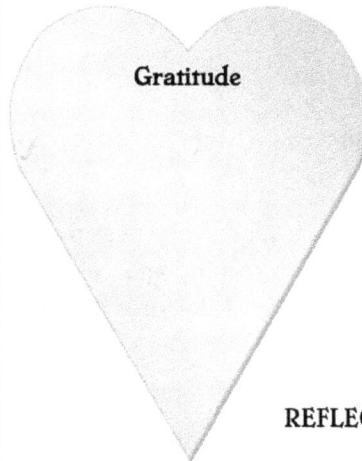

Gratitude

Food

Water: IIII IIII IIII

Breakfast:

_____
_____
_____

Lunch:

_____
_____
_____

Dinner:

_____
_____
_____

Snacks:

_____
_____
_____

Notes:

_____
_____
_____

REFLECTION

_____
_____
_____
_____
_____

Listen

I was uncomfortable over 75% of the time in my everyday life. I suffered massive cravings, headaches, panic attacks, body aches, IBS, depression. The truth was that my body was screaming for attention, but I did not want to hear what it was saying. I realize now that I was hiding from taking responsibility for my life. I can see now how clearly every piece was connected - my career, my self-esteem and my way of self-consoling with food. Once I slowed down to pay attention, it all came together.

--

Our emotions and physical symptoms are our body's messengers. Acknowledge for a moment how incredibly brilliant your body is, managing your every subconscious act from a beating heart that pumps life blood through the entirety of your being, to blinking eyes that keep those sensitive tissues moist and clear of debris. Your body works hard to manage the stress you consistently keep yourself in as it also works to use the foods you put into it for energy, building blocks, and healing.

Cravings are one of your body's messaging systems. They can be a sign of deficit or imbalance from food or from your life. If you listen to your body, this is one way to know that something is out of alignment. Other signals your body may be using include: pain, inflammation, weight loss or gain, mood swings, depression, sleeplessness, or lack of energy. Every minute your body sends signals. Are you listening to them? What is your body saying to you?

--

Try this exercise:

Take a few moments to find a comfortable seated position to settle into. Sit cross legged if on the floor, or feet on the floor if in a chair.

Take a deep breath and settle in just a little more. Close your eyes and give yourself permission to relax. Focus on your breath and notice the feeling of the breath coming and going. Notice tension you may be holding in your body and send your breath to that area to relax. Take your time to breathe and settle into this relaxation.

Draw your attention to your body as a whole. Ask yourself, "How do I feel?" Give yourself permission to hear the messages you receive. Try to receive these messages without judgement. What do you notice? What do you hear? Just notice what comes up for you and embrace it. Thank your body for the good work it does for you.

When you are ready, open your eyes and bring yourself back into your current space.

Take time to answer these questions:

What did you notice?

What sort of messages are your body sending to you?

What does this mean for you?

What might need to stay the same or change in order for you to honor the message your body is sending to you?

Next try this exercise:

Take time to listen to your body. Notice how you feel when you wake, after you eat, before you go to sleep. Check in with yourself at various times of the day. Do this throughout the next two weeks. Track what you notice in the journal pages of this workbook. At the end of the two weeks, return here to answer these questions.

What did you notice about this exercise?

How did you feel when you awoke for the day?

What did you notice about how you felt before, during, and after eating? Were you energized or exhausted after your meals? Were you satiated or over stuffed? Why did you choose to eat?

How did you feel before going to sleep?

What needs to change or stay the same in order to honor your body's messages?

DATE: _____

Morning thoughts:

_____
_____
_____
_____
_____
_____
_____

Food

Water: IIII IIII IIII

Breakfast:
_____
_____
_____

Lunch:
_____
_____
_____

Goals & Intentions for today

1
2
3
4
5
6

Dinner:
_____
_____
_____

Snacks:
_____
_____

6:00	
7:00	
8:00	
9:00	
10:00	
11:00	
12:00	
1:00	
2:00	
3:00	
4:00	
5:00	
6:00	
7:00	

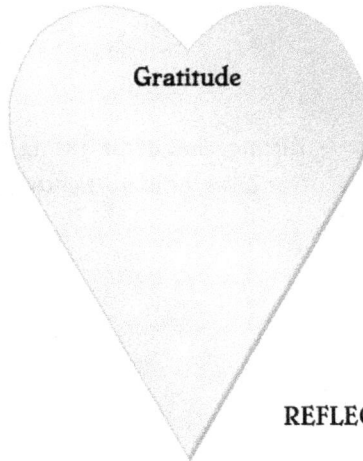

Notes:
_____
_____
_____

Gratitude

REFLECTION

_____
_____
_____
_____
_____
_____

DATE: _____

Morning thoughts:

_____
_____
_____
_____
_____
_____
_____

Goals & Intentions for today

1

2

3

4

5

6

6:00	
7:00	
8:00	
9:00	
10:00	
11:00	
12:00	
1:00	
2:00	
3:00	
4:00	
5:00	
6:00	
7:00	

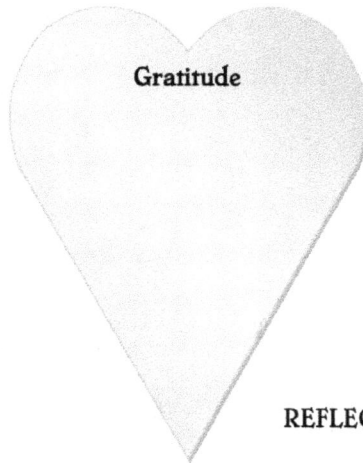

Food

Water: IIII IIII IIII

Breakfast:
_____
_____
_____

Lunch:
_____
_____
_____

Dinner:
_____
_____
_____

Snacks:
_____
_____
_____

Notes:
_____
_____
_____

Gratitude

REFLECTION

_____
_____
_____
_____
_____
_____

DATE: _____

Morning thoughts:
_____
_____
_____
_____
_____
_____
_____

Food

Water: IIII IIII IIII

Breakfast:
_____
_____
_____

Goals & Intentions for today

1
2
3
4
5
6

Lunch:
_____
_____
_____

Dinner:
_____
_____
_____

Snacks:
_____
_____

6:00	
7:00	
8:00	
9:00	
10:00	
11:00	
12:00	
1:00	
2:00	
3:00	
4:00	
5:00	
6:00	
7:00	

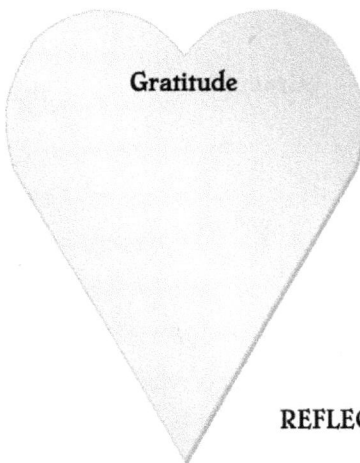

Notes:
_____
_____
_____
_____

Gratitude

REFLECTION

_____
_____
_____
_____
_____
_____

DATE: _____

Morning thoughts:
_____
_____
_____
_____
_____
_____
_____

Goals & Intentions for today

1
2
3
4
5
6

6:00	
7:00	
8:00	
9:00	
10:00	
11:00	
12:00	
1:00	
2:00	
3:00	
4:00	
5:00	
6:00	
7:00	

Food

Water: IIII IIII IIII

Breakfast:
_____
_____
_____

Lunch:
_____
_____
_____

Dinner:
_____
_____
_____

Snacks:
_____
_____

Notes:
_____
_____
_____

Gratitude

REFLECTION
_____
_____
_____
_____
_____
_____

DATE: _____

Morning thoughts:
_____
_____
_____
_____
_____
_____
_____

Food

Water: IIII IIII IIII

Breakfast:
_____
_____
_____

Goals & Intentions for today

1	
2	
3	
4	
5	
6	

Lunch:
_____
_____
_____

Dinner:
_____
_____
_____

Snacks:
_____
_____

Notes:
_____
_____
_____

6:00	
7:00	
8:00	
9:00	
10:00	
11:00	
12:00	
1:00	
2:00	
3:00	
4:00	
5:00	
6:00	
7:00	

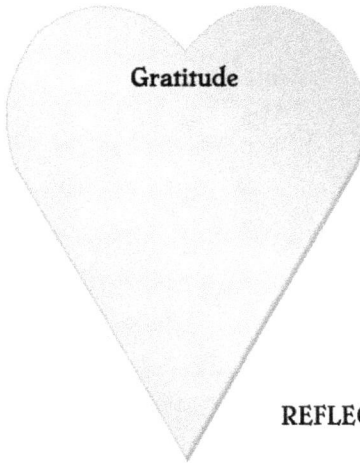

Gratitude

REFLECTION
_____
_____
_____
_____
_____
_____

DATE: _____

Morning thoughts:
_____
_____
_____
_____
_____
_____
_____

Food

Water: IIII IIII IIII

Breakfast:
_____
_____
_____

Goals & Intentions for today

1	
2	
3	
4	
5	
6	

Lunch:
_____
_____
_____

Dinner:
_____
_____
_____

Snacks:
_____
_____
_____

6:00	
7:00	
8:00	
9:00	
10:00	
11:00	
12:00	
1:00	
2:00	
3:00	
4:00	
5:00	
6:00	
7:00	

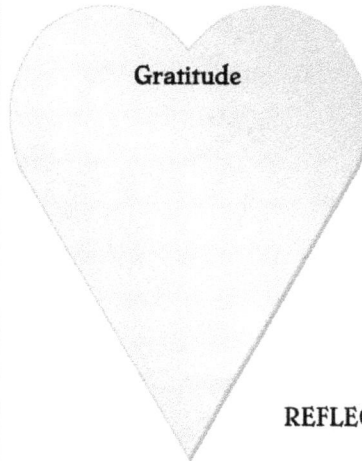

Notes:
_____
_____
_____

Gratitude

REFLECTION
_____
_____
_____
_____
_____

DATE: _____

Morning thoughts:
_____
_____
_____
_____
_____
_____
_____

Food

Water: IIII IIII IIII

Breakfast:
_____
_____

Lunch:
_____
_____
_____

Dinner:
_____
_____
_____

Snacks:
_____
_____

Notes:
_____
_____
_____
_____

Goals & Intentions for today

1
2
3
4
5
6

6:00	
7:00	
8:00	
9:00	
10:00	
11:00	
12:00	
1:00	
2:00	
3:00	
4:00	
5:00	
6:00	
7:00	

Gratitude

REFLECTION
_____
_____
_____
_____
_____
_____

DATE: _____

Morning thoughts:
_____
_____
_____
_____
_____
_____
_____

Goals & Intentions for today

1	
2	
3	
4	
5	
6	

6:00	
7:00	
8:00	
9:00	
10:00	
11:00	
12:00	
1:00	
2:00	
3:00	
4:00	
5:00	
6:00	
7:00	

Food

Water: IIII IIII IIII

Breakfast:
_____
_____
_____

Lunch:
_____
_____
_____

Dinner:
_____
_____
_____

Snacks:
_____
_____
_____

Notes:
_____
_____
_____

Gratitude

REFLECTION

_____
_____
_____
_____
_____
_____

DATE: _____

Morning thoughts:
_____
_____
_____
_____
_____
_____

Food

Water: IIII IIII IIII

Breakfast:
_____
_____
_____

Goals & Intentions for today

1
2
3
4
5
6

Lunch:
_____
_____
_____

Dinner:
_____
_____
_____

Snacks:
_____
_____
_____

6:00	
7:00	
8:00	
9:00	
10:00	
11:00	
12:00	
1:00	
2:00	
3:00	
4:00	
5:00	
6:00	
7:00	

Gratitude

Notes:
_____
_____
_____

REFLECTION

_____
_____
_____
_____
_____
_____

DATE: _____

Morning thoughts:

_____
_____
_____
_____
_____
_____
_____

Food

Water: IIII IIII IIII

Breakfast:

_____
_____
_____

Goals & Intentions for today

1	
2	
3	
4	
5	
6	

Lunch:

_____
_____
_____

Dinner:

_____
_____
_____

Snacks:

_____
_____

Notes:

_____
_____
_____
_____

6:00	
7:00	
8:00	
9:00	
10:00	
11:00	
12:00	
1:00	
2:00	
3:00	
4:00	
5:00	
6:00	
7:00	

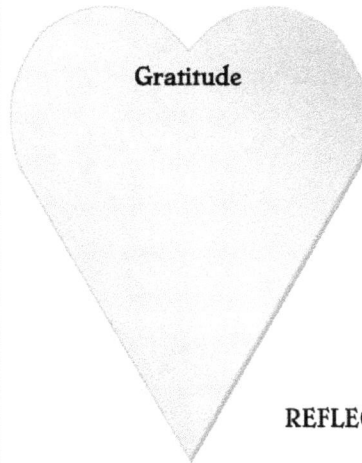

Gratitude

REFLECTION

_____
_____
_____
_____
_____

DATE: _____

Morning thoughts:
_____
_____
_____
_____
_____
_____
_____

Food

Water: IIII IIII IIII

Breakfast:
_____
_____
_____

Goals & Intentions for today

1	
2	
3	
4	
5	
6	

Lunch:
_____
_____
_____

Dinner:
_____
_____
_____

Snacks:
_____
_____

6:00	
7:00	
8:00	
9:00	
10:00	
11:00	
12:00	
1:00	
2:00	
3:00	
4:00	
5:00	
6:00	
7:00	

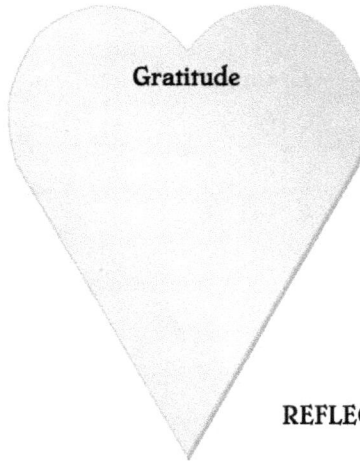

Notes:
_____
_____
_____
_____

Gratitude

REFLECTION

_____
_____
_____
_____
_____
_____

DATE: _____

Morning thoughts:
_____
_____
_____
_____
_____
_____
_____

Goals & Intentions for today

1	
2	
3	
4	
5	
6	

6:00	
7:00	
8:00	
9:00	
10:00	
11:00	
12:00	
1:00	
2:00	
3:00	
4:00	
5:00	
6:00	
7:00	

Food

Water: IIII IIII IIII

Breakfast:
_____
_____
_____

Lunch:
_____
_____
_____

Dinner:
_____
_____
_____

Snacks:
_____
_____

Notes:
_____
_____
_____

Gratitude

REFLECTION
_____
_____
_____
_____
_____
_____

DATE: _____

Morning thoughts:
_____
_____
_____
_____
_____
_____
_____

Food

Water: IIII IIII IIII

Breakfast:
_____
_____
_____

Goals & Intentions for today

1
2
3
4
5
6

Lunch:
_____
_____
_____

Dinner:
_____
_____

Snacks:
_____
_____

6:00	
7:00	
8:00	
9:00	
10:00	
11:00	
12:00	
1:00	
2:00	
3:00	
4:00	
5:00	
6:00	
7:00	

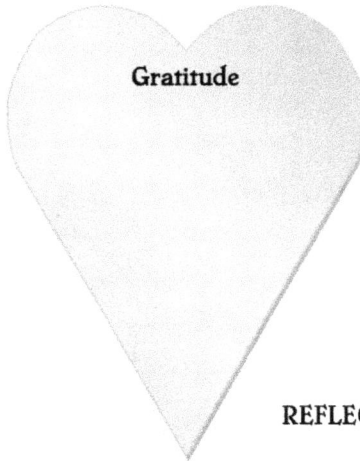

Notes:
_____
_____
_____

Gratitude

REFLECTION

_____
_____
_____
_____
_____
_____

DATE: _____

Morning thoughts:

_____
_____
_____
_____
_____
_____
_____

Food

Water: IIII IIII IIII

Breakfast:

_____
_____
_____

Lunch:

_____
_____
_____

Dinner:

_____
_____
_____

Snacks:

_____
_____
_____

Notes:

_____
_____
_____

Goals & Intentions for today

1	
2	
3	
4	
5	
6	

6:00	
7:00	
8:00	
9:00	
10:00	
11:00	
12:00	
1:00	
2:00	
3:00	
4:00	
5:00	
6:00	
7:00	

Gratitude

REFLECTION

_____
_____
_____
_____
_____
_____

Move

In my younger years, I was very active. We lived in the country and I have so many memories climbing trees, digging, catching frogs and collecting pine cones. When we moved to Denver, the wilderness play turned to kickball, soft ball, and even flag football with the neighborhood boys. As I grew, my interests varied from dancing to gymnastics. As a young adult, I loved to go clubbing a few nights every week. All the activity kept my body strong and lean well into my twenties.

Then, I met my now husband and I both literally and figuratively settled down. I pushed aside movement as I knew it. While we would go for the occasional hike or bike ride, most of the time we were focused on home building projects and our careers. Really, building the lives we have today.

As I entered my thirties, I tried to get a grip on my increasing weight and I re-immersed myself into movement. I'd walk on work breaks, go to the gym at lunch with friends, eventually graduating to my beloved Pilates and yoga. These were the most satisfying for me.

——

Movement plays an important role in your self-care plans especially today since we are up against society norms that are more sedentary than ever before.

More people have desk jobs often for up to 10 hours a day. This is followed by a long seated stressful commute. Meals are often seated and followed by an evening filled with seated relaxation. Our bodies were not made for so much sitting.

Like food, movement is very personal. This is called Bio-individuality™, which means simply, the answer is inside *you*. We are all truly unique beings. Some thrive on high impact, plyometric, cross fit, or weight lifting. Others find their answer through running, jumping rope, Zumba, or aerobics. Still others are most satisfied and healthy with meditative calming Pilates, yoga, or walking. The best way to know what will work for you is to experiment with it in your every day life.

Movement goes far beyond structured exercise. It can mean walking your dog around the block, playing with your kids, and parking further from the store. It can mean taking the stairs instead of the elevator, or hiking in the woods. It can mean all of these things, or just one.

Tips to increase movement every day:

Tools that make it easier:

Pedometer or a Smart Band – like a Fitbit
Exercise Journal
Weights
Stretch Bands
Yoga Mat
Water Bottle
Good Tennis Shoes

Ways to fit it in:

Join a club, gym, or class
Get a trainer
Find a nature center to explore
Play interactive video games, like Kinect
Play chase or ball with your kids
Walk your dog
Take walking breaks at work

Take some time to answer these questions:

1. What sort of movement do you already include in your everyday life?

2. How much time do you move?

3. How much time do you sit?

4. What forms of exercise have you tried in the past?

5. How did they feel for you?

6. Have you stopped them? Why?

7. What new movement or exercise would you like to try?

TAKE ACTION & SCHEDULE IT!

Try this exercise:

Look at your planner for the next two weeks. Find 30 minutes in each day that you can block out specifically for movement. What this looks like is completely up to you – you can do this in the morning or evening, or even on your lunch break.

Choose a single form of exercise that you will do in this 30 minute time frame.

At the end of the two weeks answer the following questions:

1. Did you follow through with your plan?

2. What exercise did you choose?

3. How was it for you? What would you like to do differently?

4. What is the next form of movement or exercise you'll try?

P.S. As a busy mom, I know how hard it might be to prioritize movement. I choose 30 minutes every week day morning as my focused exercise time. I might use a video, my treadmill, or elliptical during this time. Then I focus movement on life for the rest of the day. I keep the television off and make sure I'm up doing chores and playing with my son. We walk together, swim together, do yard work together, and play together. All movement counts. The more you do, the better you will feel!

Journal & Schedule

Morning thoughts:
_____
_____
_____
_____
_____
_____
_____

Goals & Intentions for today

1
2
3
4
5
6

6:00	
7:00	
8:00	
9:00	
10:00	
11:00	
12:00	
1:00	
2:00	
3:00	
4:00	
5:00	
6:00	
7:00	

Food

Water: IIII IIII IIII

Breakfast:
_____
_____
_____

Lunch:
_____
_____
_____

Dinner:
_____
_____
_____

Snacks:
_____
_____

Notes:
_____
_____
_____

Gratitude

REFLECTION
_____
_____
_____
_____
_____
_____

DATE: _____

Morning thoughts:
_____
_____
_____
_____
_____
_____
_____

Goals & Intentions for today

1	
2	
3	
4	
5	
6	

6:00	
7:00	
8:00	
9:00	
10:00	
11:00	
12:00	
1:00	
2:00	
3:00	
4:00	
5:00	
6:00	
7:00	

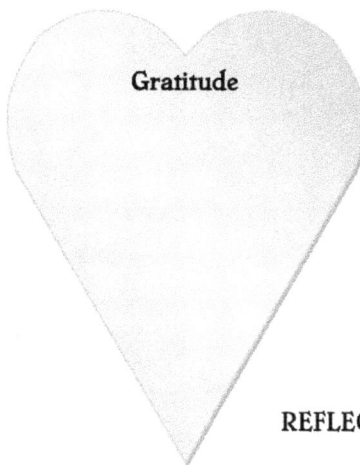

Gratitude

Food

Water: IIII IIII IIII

Breakfast:
_____
_____
_____

Lunch:
_____
_____
_____

Dinner:
_____
_____
_____

Snacks:
_____
_____
_____

Notes:
_____
_____
_____

REFLECTION

_____
_____
_____
_____
_____
_____

DATE: _____

Morning thoughts:
_____
_____
_____
_____
_____
_____
_____

Food

Water: IIII IIII IIII

Breakfast:
_____
_____
_____

Lunch:
_____
_____
_____

Dinner:
_____
_____
_____

Snacks:
_____
_____
_____

Notes:
_____
_____
_____

Goals & Intentions for today

1
2
3
4
5
6

6:00	
7:00	
8:00	
9:00	
10:00	
11:00	
12:00	
1:00	
2:00	
3:00	
4:00	
5:00	
6:00	
7:00	

Gratitude

REFLECTION
_____
_____
_____
_____
_____
_____

DATE: _____

Morning thoughts:
_____
_____
_____
_____
_____
_____
_____

Goals & Intentions for today

1
2
3
4
5
6

6:00	
7:00	
8:00	
9:00	
10:00	
11:00	
12:00	
1:00	
2:00	
3:00	
4:00	
5:00	
6:00	
7:00	

Food

Water: IIII IIII IIII

Breakfast:
_____
_____
_____

Lunch:
_____
_____
_____

Dinner:
_____
_____
_____

Snacks:
_____
_____

Notes:
_____
_____
_____

Gratitude

REFLECTION
_____
_____
_____
_____
_____
_____

DATE: _____

Morning thoughts:
_____
_____
_____
_____
_____
_____
_____

Food

Water: IIII IIII IIII

Breakfast:
_____
_____
_____

Goals & Intentions for today

1

2

3

Lunch:
_____
_____
_____

4

5

6

Dinner:
_____
_____
_____

Snacks:
_____
_____

6:00	
7:00	
8:00	
9:00	
10:00	
11:00	
12:00	
1:00	
2:00	
3:00	
4:00	
5:00	
6:00	
7:00	

Notes:
_____
_____
_____

Gratitude

REFLECTION

_____
_____
_____
_____
_____
_____

Journal & Schedule

Morning thoughts:

_____
_____
_____
_____
_____
_____
_____

Food

Water: IIII IIII IIII

Breakfast:
_____
_____
_____

Lunch:
_____
_____
_____

Dinner:
_____
_____
_____

Snacks:
_____
_____
_____

Notes:
_____
_____
_____

Goals & Intentions for today

1
2
3
4
5
6

6:00	
7:00	
8:00	
9:00	
10:00	
11:00	
12:00	
1:00	
2:00	
3:00	
4:00	
5:00	
6:00	
7:00	

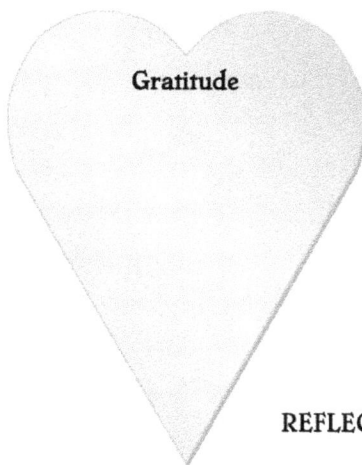

Gratitude

REFLECTION

_____
_____
_____
_____
_____
_____

DATE: _____

Morning thoughts:
_____
_____
_____
_____
_____
_____
_____

Food

Water: IIII IIII IIII

Breakfast:
_____
_____
_____

Lunch:
_____
_____
_____

Goals & Intentions for today

1	
2	
3	
4	
5	
6	

Dinner:
_____
_____
_____

Snacks:
_____
_____

Notes:
_____

6:00	
7:00	
8:00	
9:00	
10:00	
11:00	
12:00	
1:00	
2:00	
3:00	
4:00	
5:00	
6:00	
7:00	

Gratitude

_____
_____

REFLECTION

_____
_____
_____
_____
_____
_____

DATE: _____

Morning thoughts:
_____
_____
_____
_____
_____
_____
_____

Goals & Intentions for today

1
2
3
4
5
6

Food

Water: IIII IIII IIII

Breakfast:
_____
_____
_____

Lunch:
_____
_____
_____

Dinner:
_____
_____
_____

Snacks:
_____
_____
_____

Notes:
_____
_____
_____

6:00	
7:00	
8:00	
9:00	
10:00	
11:00	
12:00	
1:00	
2:00	
3:00	
4:00	
5:00	
6:00	
7:00	

Gratitude

REFLECTION
_____
_____
_____
_____
_____
_____

DATE: _____

Morning thoughts:
_____
_____
_____
_____
_____
_____
_____

Goals & Intentions for today

1
2
3
4
5
6

6:00	
7:00	
8:00	
9:00	
10:00	
11:00	
12:00	
1:00	
2:00	
3:00	
4:00	
5:00	
6:00	
7:00	

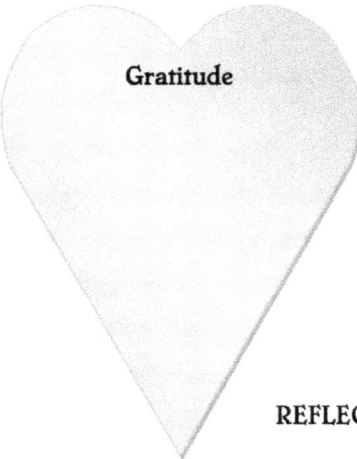

Food

Water: IIII IIII IIII

Breakfast:
_____
_____
_____

Lunch:
_____
_____
_____

Dinner:
_____
_____
_____

Snacks:
_____
_____

Notes:
_____
_____
_____

Gratitude

REFLECTION

_____
_____
_____
_____
_____
_____

DATE: _____

Journal & Schedule

Morning thoughts:
_____
_____
_____
_____
_____
_____
_____

Food

Water: IIII IIII IIII

Breakfast:
_____
_____
_____

Goals & Intentions for today

1	
2	
3	
4	
5	
6	

Lunch:
_____
_____
_____

Dinner:
_____
_____
_____

Snacks:
_____
_____

6:00	
7:00	
8:00	
9:00	
10:00	
11:00	
12:00	
1:00	
2:00	
3:00	
4:00	
5:00	
6:00	
7:00	

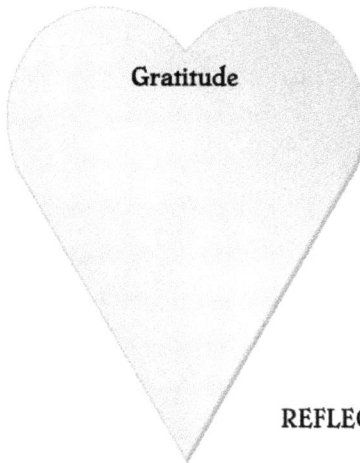

Notes:
_____
_____
_____
_____

Gratitude

REFLECTION

_____
_____
_____
_____
_____
_____

DATE: _____

Morning thoughts:
_____
_____
_____
_____
_____
_____
_____

Goals & Intentions for today

1
2
3
4
5
6

6:00	
7:00	
8:00	
9:00	
10:00	
11:00	
12:00	
1:00	
2:00	
3:00	
4:00	
5:00	
6:00	
7:00	

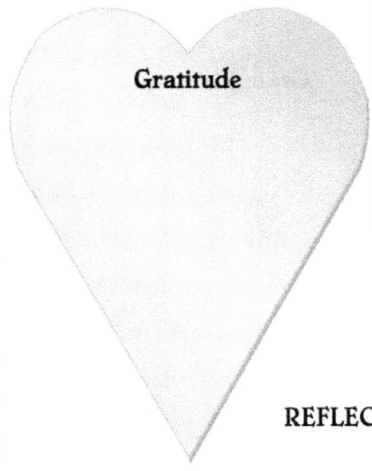

Food

Water: IIII IIII IIII

Breakfast:
_____
_____
_____

Lunch:
_____
_____
_____

Dinner:
_____
_____
_____

Snacks:
_____
_____
_____

Notes:
_____
_____
_____

Gratitude

REFLECTION
_____
_____
_____
_____
_____
_____

DATE: _____

Morning thoughts:
_____
_____
_____
_____
_____
_____
_____

Food

Water: IIII IIII IIII

Breakfast:
_____
_____
_____

Goals & Intentions for today

1	
2	
3	
4	
5	
6	

Lunch:
_____
_____
_____

Dinner:
_____
_____
_____

Snacks:
_____
_____

6:00	
7:00	
8:00	
9:00	
10:00	
11:00	
12:00	
1:00	
2:00	
3:00	
4:00	
5:00	
6:00	
7:00	

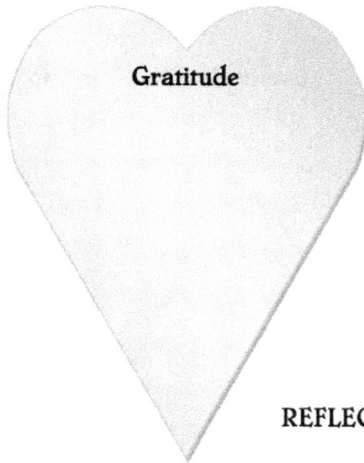

Gratitude

Notes:
_____
_____
_____

REFLECTION

_____
_____
_____
_____
_____
_____

DATE: _____

Morning thoughts:
_____
_____
_____
_____
_____
_____

Goals & Intentions for today

1	
2	
3	
4	
5	
6	

6:00	
7:00	
8:00	
9:00	
10:00	
11:00	
12:00	
1:00	
2:00	
3:00	
4:00	
5:00	
6:00	
7:00	

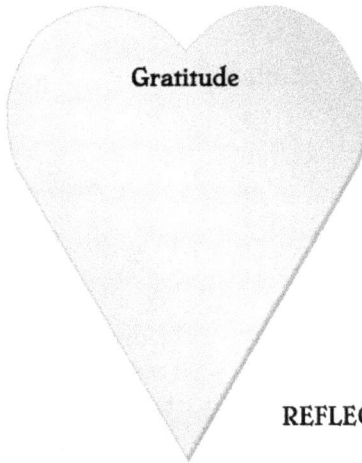

Food

Water: IIII IIII IIII

Breakfast:
_____
_____
_____

Lunch:
_____
_____
_____

Dinner:
_____
_____
_____

Snacks:
_____
_____

Notes:
_____
_____
_____
_____

Gratitude

REFLECTION
_____
_____
_____
_____
_____
_____

126

DATE: _____

Morning thoughts:

_____
_____
_____
_____
_____
_____
_____

Goals & Intentions for today

1	
2	
3	
4	
5	
6	

6:00	
7:00	
8:00	
9:00	
10:00	
11:00	
12:00	
1:00	
2:00	
3:00	
4:00	
5:00	
6:00	
7:00	

Food

Water: IIII IIII IIII

Breakfast:
_____
_____
_____

Lunch:
_____
_____
_____

Dinner:
_____
_____
_____

Snacks:
_____
_____
_____

Notes:
_____
_____
_____

Gratitude

REFLECTION

_____
_____
_____
_____
_____
_____

Sleep

My mind spins with thoughts. Laying, in the dark, eyes closed, I am replaying the events of the day. I can't get past it. The stress mounds. I replay it again.

Without resolution, I lay in bed for hours thinking about any stressful moment my mind can grab onto, turning it over and over. Sometimes, my mind will begin to wander and allow a few other thoughts to invade. I'll drift, then remember. I lay awake wishing I could go to sleep.

The next day, I'm in a fog. I have very little energy and I'm not thinking clearly. The stressful moments I was ruminating on the night before feel magnified and heavy. I want to cry, and I want to sleep.

--

A good night's sleep might make all the difference in the world but there may be many reasons why sleep can be evasive or disrupted: busy mind, too much caffeine, not enough movement throughout the day, not enough natural light, physical pain, dehydration, exposure to television or computer screens too close to bed time or maybe even a combination of these things.

Lack of quality sleep can interfere with emotions, memory, focus, energy, and even long term health. Often those who don't sleep well talk about having an increase in food cravings. Sleep is a time for restoration and renewal, emotionally and physically. Depriving yourself of this much needed time will certainly affect your ability to meet your wellness goals.

Tips to improve your sleep:

- ∞ Reduce or eliminate your daily caffeine intake.
  - o If you love coffee, try cutting back gently by replacing half of your blend with decaf, or trading out a cup with a decaffeinated coffee replacement or alternative like Teeccino.
- ∞ Unplug at least an hour before bed.
  - o If you like to read at bed time, opt for either a paper book rather than an eBook, or alter the brightness of your device manually or via an app.
- ∞ Don't eat within an hour of bed time.
- ∞ Get outside every day to expose yourself to natural light. Our circadian rhythm is activated and ruled through our eyes.
- ∞ Give yourself time to decompress.
- ∞ Develop a routine with one or all of the above. Having a repeated routine allows your body and mind to know what to expect and thus, relax into it.
- ∞ Journal your thoughts and events from the day.
- ∞ Keep a gratitude journal.

P.S. Children thrive on routine. If you aren't sleeping because your children aren't sleeping, consider checking in with all of these same ideas. Be cautious with sugar after dinner, reducing all forms of sugar including juice, fruit, and bread.

Try this exercise:

In the journal pages of this book, log your sleep for the next two weeks and notice your sleep quality, bed time habits, and evening routines. Try to bring awareness to food and drink consumed within a few hours of bedtime. For some, this can be a sleep inhibitor. If you use a Fitbit or other device that tracks your sleep, make note of waking and restless times. At the end of the two weeks, answer the following questions.

1. How are you sleeping?

2. What do you notice about your bed time routines?

3. Are there lifestyle factors that may be playing a role in your sleep quality? If so, which ones? What feels like it's working well?

4. What types of changes do you need to make in order to improve your sleep?

5. How do you feel when you have *not* had a good night's sleep?

6. How do you feel when you are fully rested?

TAKE ACTION & SCHEDULE IT!

Choose a time in the evening to begin to settle down for the night. Set a reminder on your smart phone or computer to unplug at least 50 minutes before this time. Honor it.

"My diet was improved without ever feeling like I was on a diet. I naturally want to eat the way I eat now, my old cravings and poor habits went away seemingly on their own! Tammi has helped me shift my entire life into a more well-balanced, healthy lifestyle." – Sarah M.

K.I.S.S. (Keep It Simple Silly!)

Vegan, Gluten Free, Dairy Free, Celiac, Nutritarian, Paleo, Atkins, Lacto-Ovo Vegetarian, Nut Free, High Carb, Low Carb, No Carb - the list goes on and on. In fact, there are hundreds of dietary theories floating around in the world today. Everyone it seems, has an idea of what the perfect diet is. Unfortunately, no one diet is the perfect diet for everyone. Chances are, that is why you are here in the first place. It's not to remember to breathe, or to add more movement into your everyday life. It's to figure out exactly what the magic combination of foods are for your body – that one magical formula that allows you to find your perfect, balanced, happy, body.

I've created this portion of my workbook to help you begin to decode this part of your health and wellbeing. Essentially, to remind you of what you know so well already. One step at a time, I'll introduce you to ideas about food and habits around it that will help you to uncover what works for you. What I won't be doing is giving you an over complicated restrictive diet plan. In fact, we'll be working together to keep it really, really simple.

A few tips to remember as you work through this portion of the MomPositive Workbook:

1. **You are a completely, magnificently, unique being.** Just because it's written here doesn't mean it will be a guaranteed fit for you. This is about experimenting and finding what will work, what feels good, learning to listen and to honor that. There are factors outside those that I mention in this workbook. Feel free to add more topics to your experimentation as you go and if you need my support, reach out to me for a complimentary consultation.
2. **There are no hard steadfast rules.** Our physical and emotional needs change as our lifestyle, stress levels, physical work load, and hormones change. This is about learning to listen to your body – not to develop unbreakable rules.
3. **Making changes in eating habits can take time.** The cool thing is that you have this guide. If you fall off of a routine that was working for you, come back here, revisit your journey, and get back on track.
4. **We all make mistakes, not one of us is perfect, and it's perfectly okay to own that part of you.** Being healthy is a life long journey. There is no end point or destination. Every single day, we must make a renewed commitment to the journey.
5. **Know and embrace that you will live a more fulfilled, healthy, and happy life because of these healthy choices you are making.** Celebrate every single step!
6. **Use the planner to work for you.** Time management and learning to prioritize our wellbeing is the number one block for all of my clients. For some, this means sitting with your planner weekly, mapping out your game plan, and setting down details. For others, it's a nightly routine, – identifying your intentions based on reflections from the day. Whatever works for you is fine.
7. **Track your food.** Remember, doing so increases your chances of success.
8. **Get more support if you need it.** Look around you – who can support you in your life? A family member? A friend? An Integrative Nutrition Health Coach™? A doctor? A therapist?

DATE: _____

Journal & Schedule

Morning thoughts:

_____
_____
_____
_____
_____
_____
_____

Goals & Intentions for today

1
2
3
4
5
6

6:00	
7:00	
8:00	
9:00	
10:00	
11:00	
12:00	
1:00	
2:00	
3:00	
4:00	
5:00	
6:00	
7:00	

Gratitude

Food

Water: IIII IIII IIII

Breakfast:
_____
_____
_____

Lunch:
_____
_____
_____

Dinner:
_____
_____
_____

Snacks:
_____
_____

Notes:
_____
_____
_____
_____

REFLECTION

_____
_____
_____
_____
_____
_____

DATE: _____

Morning thoughts:
_____
_____
_____
_____
_____
_____
_____

Goals & Intentions for today

1
2
3
4
5
6

6:00	
7:00	
8:00	
9:00	
10:00	
11:00	
12:00	
1:00	
2:00	
3:00	
4:00	
5:00	
6:00	
7:00	

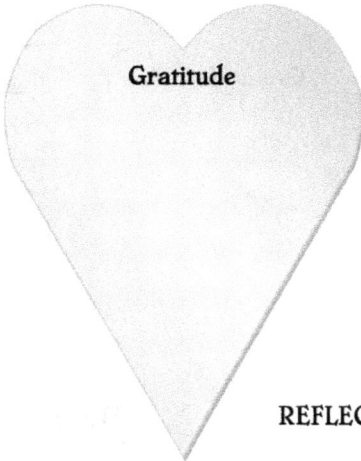

Food

Water: IIII IIII IIII

Breakfast:
_____
_____
_____

Lunch:
_____
_____
_____

Dinner:
_____
_____
_____

Snacks:
_____
_____

Notes:
_____
_____
_____

Gratitude

REFLECTION
_____
_____
_____
_____
_____

DATE: _____

Morning thoughts:
_____
_____
_____
_____
_____
_____
_____

Food

Water: IIII IIII IIII

Breakfast:
_____
_____
_____

Goals & Intentions for today

1	
2	
3	
4	
5	
6	

Lunch:
_____
_____
_____

Dinner:
_____
_____
_____

Snacks:
_____
_____

Notes:
_____
_____
_____

6:00	
7:00	
8:00	
9:00	
10:00	
11:00	
12:00	
1:00	
2:00	
3:00	
4:00	
5:00	
6:00	
7:00	

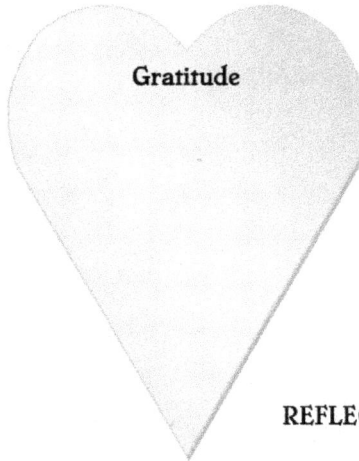

Gratitude

REFLECTION
_____
_____
_____
_____
_____
_____

DATE: _____

Morning thoughts:
_____
_____
_____
_____
_____
_____
_____

Goals & Intentions for today

1
2
3
4
5
6

6:00	
7:00	
8:00	
9:00	
10:00	
11:00	
12:00	
1:00	
2:00	
3:00	
4:00	
5:00	
6:00	
7:00	

Food

Water: IIII IIII IIII

Breakfast:
_____
_____
_____

Lunch:
_____
_____
_____

Dinner:
_____
_____
_____

Snacks:
_____
_____
_____

Notes:
_____
_____
_____

Gratitude

REFLECTION
_____
_____
_____
_____
_____
_____

DATE: _____

Morning thoughts:
_____
_____
_____
_____
_____
_____
_____

Food

Water: IIII IIII IIII

Breakfast:
_____
_____

Goals & Intentions for today

| 1 |
| 2 |
| 3 |
| 4 |
| 5 |
| 6 |

Lunch:
_____
_____
_____

Dinner:
_____
_____
_____

Snacks:
_____
_____

Notes:
_____
_____
_____

6:00	
7:00	
8:00	
9:00	
10:00	
11:00	
12:00	
1:00	
2:00	
3:00	
4:00	
5:00	
6:00	
7:00	

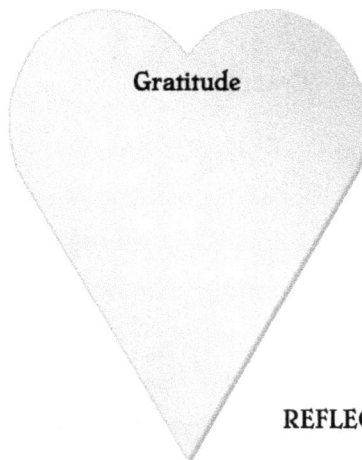

Gratitude

REFLECTION
_____
_____
_____
_____
_____
_____

Morning thoughts:
_____
_____
_____
_____
_____
_____
_____
_____

Goals & Intentions for today

1
2
3
4
5
6

6:00	
7:00	
8:00	
9:00	
10:00	
11:00	
12:00	
1:00	
2:00	
3:00	
4:00	
5:00	
6:00	
7:00	

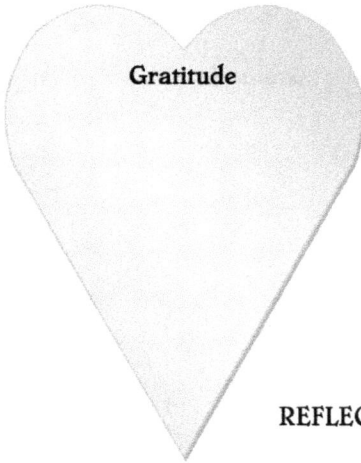

Food

Water: IIII IIII IIII

Breakfast:
_____
_____
_____

Lunch:
_____
_____
_____

Dinner:
_____
_____
_____

Snacks:
_____
_____

Notes:
_____
_____
_____

Journal & Schedule

Gratitude

REFLECTION
_____
_____
_____
_____
_____
_____

DATE: _____

Morning thoughts:
_____
_____
_____
_____
_____
_____

Food

Water: IIII IIII IIII

Breakfast:
_____
_____
_____

Goals & Intentions for today

1	
2	
3	
4	
5	
6	

Lunch:
_____
_____
_____

Dinner:
_____
_____

Snacks:
_____
_____

6:00	
7:00	
8:00	
9:00	
10:00	
11:00	
12:00	
1:00	
2:00	
3:00	
4:00	
5:00	
6:00	
7:00	

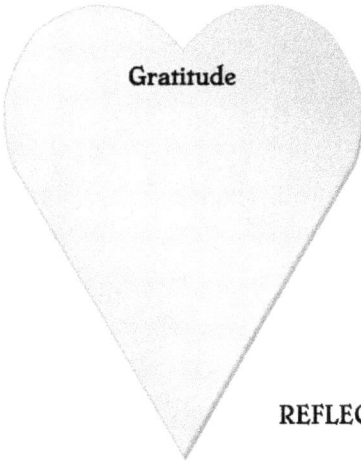

Notes:
_____
_____
_____

Gratitude

REFLECTION
_____
_____
_____
_____
_____
_____

138

DATE: _____

Morning thoughts:
_____
_____
_____
_____
_____
_____
_____

Goals & Intentions for today

1	
2	
3	
4	
5	
6	

6:00	
7:00	
8:00	
9:00	
10:00	
11:00	
12:00	
1:00	
2:00	
3:00	
4:00	
5:00	
6:00	
7:00	

Food

Water: IIII IIII IIII

Breakfast:
_____
_____
_____

Lunch:
_____
_____
_____

Dinner:
_____
_____
_____

Snacks:
_____
_____

Notes:
_____
_____
_____
_____

Gratitude

REFLECTION
_____
_____
_____
_____
_____
_____

Journal & Schedule

Morning thoughts:
_____
_____
_____
_____
_____
_____
_____
_____

Food

Water: IIII IIII IIII

Breakfast:
_____
_____
_____

Goals & Intentions for today

1	
2	
3	
4	
5	
6	

Lunch:
_____
_____
_____

Dinner:
_____
_____
_____

Snacks:
_____
_____
_____

6:00	
7:00	
8:00	
9:00	
10:00	
11:00	
12:00	
1:00	
2:00	
3:00	
4:00	
5:00	
6:00	
7:00	

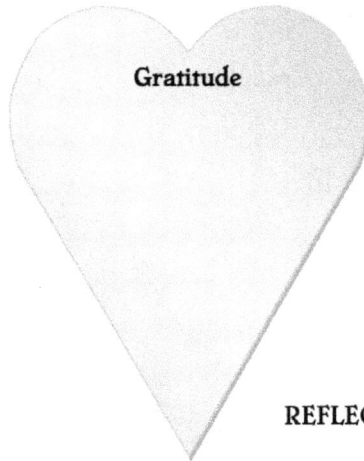

Gratitude

Notes:
_____
_____
_____
_____

REFLECTION

_____
_____
_____
_____
_____
_____

DATE: _____

Morning thoughts:
_____
_____
_____
_____
_____
_____
_____

Goals & Intentions for today

1
2
3
4
5
6

6:00	
7:00	
8:00	
9:00	
10:00	
11:00	
12:00	
1:00	
2:00	
3:00	
4:00	
5:00	
6:00	
7:00	

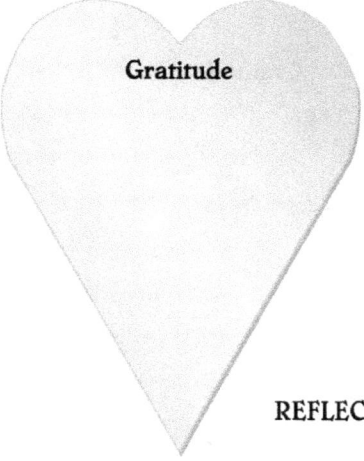

Food

Water: IIII IIII IIII

Breakfast:
_____
_____
_____

Lunch:
_____
_____
_____

Dinner:
_____
_____
_____

Snacks:
_____
_____

Notes:
_____
_____
_____

Gratitude

REFLECTION

_____
_____
_____
_____
_____
_____

DATE: _____

Morning thoughts:
_____
_____
_____
_____
_____
_____
_____

Food

Water: IIII IIII IIII

Breakfast:
_____
_____
_____

Goals & Intentions for today

1	
2	
3	
4	
5	
6	

Lunch:
_____
_____
_____

Dinner:
_____
_____
_____

Snacks:
_____
_____

6:00	
7:00	
8:00	
9:00	
10:00	
11:00	
12:00	
1:00	
2:00	
3:00	
4:00	
5:00	
6:00	
7:00	

Gratitude

Notes:
_____
_____
_____

REFLECTION

_____
_____
_____
_____
_____
_____

DATE: _____

Morning thoughts:

_____
_____
_____
_____
_____
_____
_____

Food

Water: IIII IIII IIII

Breakfast:
_____
_____
_____

Goals & Intentions for today

1	
2	
3	
4	
5	
6	

Lunch:
_____
_____
_____

Dinner:
_____
_____
_____

Snacks:
_____
_____

6:00	
7:00	
8:00	
9:00	
10:00	
11:00	
12:00	
1:00	
2:00	
3:00	
4:00	
5:00	
6:00	
7:00	

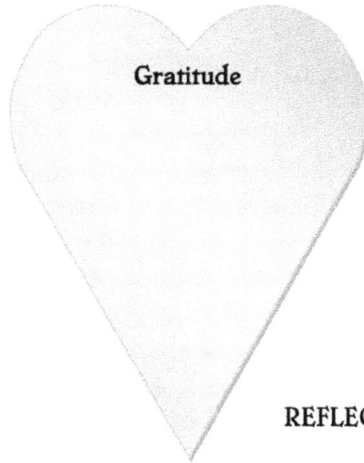

Notes:
_____
_____
_____

Gratitude

REFLECTION

_____
_____
_____
_____
_____
_____

DATE: _____

Morning thoughts:
_____
_____
_____
_____
_____
_____
_____

Food

Water: IIII IIII IIII

Breakfast:
_____
_____
_____

Goals & Intentions for today

1	
2	
3	
4	
5	
6	

Lunch:
_____
_____
_____

Dinner:
_____
_____
_____

Snacks:
_____
_____

6:00	
7:00	
8:00	
9:00	
10:00	
11:00	
12:00	
1:00	
2:00	
3:00	
4:00	
5:00	
6:00	
7:00	

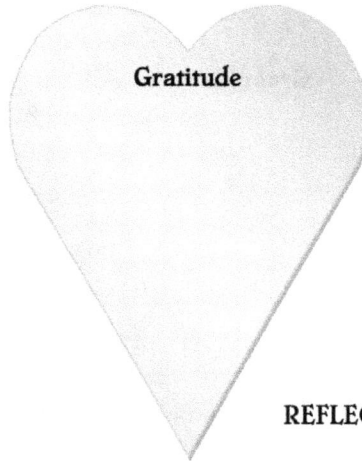

Gratitude

Notes:
_____
_____
_____

REFLECTION

_____
_____
_____
_____
_____
_____

DATE: _____

Morning thoughts:

_____
_____
_____
_____
_____
_____
_____

Goals & Intentions for today

1
2
3
4
5
6

6:00	
7:00	
8:00	
9:00	
10:00	
11:00	
12:00	
1:00	
2:00	
3:00	
4:00	
5:00	
6:00	
7:00	

Food

Water: IIII IIII IIII

Breakfast:
_____
_____

Lunch:
_____
_____
_____

Dinner:
_____
_____
_____

Snacks:
_____
_____

Notes:
_____
_____
_____
_____

Gratitude

REFLECTION

_____
_____
_____
_____
_____

Eat Clean

"Let food be thy medicine and thy medicine be thy food" – Hippocrates

In my first year of learning how to take care of this body of mine, I watched for and selected more foods that made health claims such as, "High in fiber!" and "More Calcium than a glass of milk!" I swallowed more supplements than food, and drank massive amounts of sports drinks and protein shakes. I also gained a lot of weight and felt really terrible despite working out over an hour every day, plus my daily two mile walk.

It was frightening, frustrating, and overwhelming to keep going forward. It was during this time that I realized I had no idea how to take care of my own body. It was quite an awakening.

--

The Rules for Eating Clean

1. **Choose foods in their most natural form.** Avoid, reduce, and minimize any food that is processed or boxed.
2. **See rule #1.**

I could add or make up a lot of additional rules here but I prefer not to. (Remember K.I.S.S.?) Bottom line, it's about going back to natural food. If you eat whole foods, you naturally avoid chemicalized, artificial and unnatural junk food that our body cannot effectively use as building material or for energy.

The easiest way to do this? Eat food that looks like, well....., *FOOD!*

--

As a society, we are generally over fed and under nourished. Most of the items we put in our mouths (and our unsuspecting children's mouths), are completely processed, nutrient void, chemical laden, nonfood substances.

As you add more real food to your plate, you will naturally push away those things that are less nourishing. This is an idea called "crowding out". Instead of saying – "No, you cannot have that soda"; we say, "drink herbal tea first."

Instead of restricting, we simply replace.

Choices that fit into the Clean Foods category include: carrots, mushrooms, greens, apples, endive, chard, sprouts, beets, cabbage, peppers, tomatoes, grapes, lettuce, arugula, radishes, chives, onions, leeks, potatoes, squash, beans, and berries. There are far too many to list here, but you get the idea. Of course, this includes meats like fish, pasture raised chicken, pasture raised beef, pasture raised pork, or other high quality, naturally raised and butchered meats.

Each one of these foods has a phenomenally different nutrient profile that works synergistically with your body to build strength and provide a foundation for health.

Try this exercise:

Take a few minutes to visit your kitchen. Notice every food item that you have that follows the Eat Clean rules.

Now notice those items that don't follow the Eat Clean rules. Try not to judge, just notice.

Pick one or two whole foods that you'd like to add to your Eat Clean options and write it here.

TAKE ACTION & SCHEDULE IT!

When will you start? Write the date in your planner.

Where will you get it?

How will you prepare it? (Recipe, raw, salad...)

After you've done this exercise, write down how it went. Include what you'd like to do the same or differently next time. What do you notice about the foods, choices, and preparation?

What is your goal with eating clean?

How frequently would you like to include a whole food in your diet? Daily? Weekly?

"You don't have to be great to start, but you have to start to be great!" – Zig Ziglar

DATE: _____

Morning thoughts:
_____
_____
_____
_____
_____
_____
_____

Goals & Intentions for today

1	
2	
3	
4	
5	
6	

6:00	
7:00	
8:00	
9:00	
10:00	
11:00	
12:00	
1:00	
2:00	
3:00	
4:00	
5:00	
6:00	
7:00	

Gratitude

Food

Water: IIII IIII IIII

Breakfast:
_____
_____
_____

Lunch:
_____
_____
_____

Dinner:
_____
_____
_____

Snacks:
_____
_____
_____

Notes:
_____
_____
_____

REFLECTION

_____
_____
_____
_____
_____

DATE: _____

Morning thoughts:
_____
_____
_____
_____
_____
_____
_____

Food

Water: IIII IIII IIII

Breakfast:
_____
_____
_____

Goals & Intentions for today

1
2
3
4
5
6

Lunch:
_____
_____
_____

Dinner:
_____
_____
_____

Snacks:
_____
_____

6:00	
7:00	
8:00	
9:00	
10:00	
11:00	
12:00	
1:00	
2:00	
3:00	
4:00	
5:00	
6:00	
7:00	

Notes:
_____
_____
_____

Gratitude

REFLECTION

_____
_____
_____
_____
_____

DATE: _____

Morning thoughts:
_____
_____
_____
_____
_____
_____
_____

Food

Water: IIII IIII IIII

Breakfast:
_____
_____
_____

Lunch:
_____
_____
_____

Goals & Intentions for today

1

2

3

4

5

6

Dinner:
_____
_____
_____

Snacks:
_____
_____

6:00	
7:00	
8:00	
9:00	
10:00	
11:00	
12:00	
1:00	
2:00	
3:00	
4:00	
5:00	
6:00	
7:00	

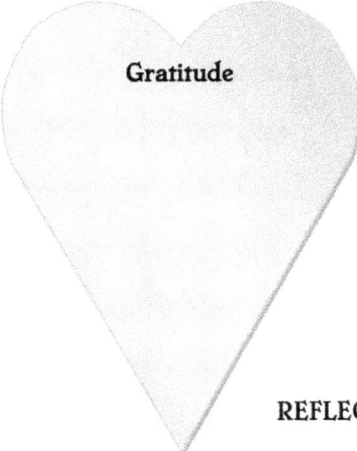

Gratitude

Notes:
_____
_____
_____

REFLECTION

_____
_____
_____
_____
_____
_____

DATE: _____

Morning thoughts:
_____
_____
_____
_____
_____
_____
_____

Goals & Intentions for today

1	
2	
3	
4	
5	
6	

6:00	
7:00	
8:00	
9:00	
10:00	
11:00	
12:00	
1:00	
2:00	
3:00	
4:00	
5:00	
6:00	
7:00	

Food

Water: IIII IIII IIII

Breakfast:
_____
_____

Lunch:
_____
_____
_____

Dinner:
_____
_____
_____

Snacks:
_____
_____

Notes:
_____
_____
_____

Gratitude

REFLECTION
_____
_____
_____
_____
_____
_____

Journal & Schedule

Morning thoughts:
_____
_____
_____
_____
_____
_____
_____

Goals & Intentions for today

1
2
3
4
5
6

6:00	
7:00	
8:00	
9:00	
10:00	
11:00	
12:00	
1:00	
2:00	
3:00	
4:00	
5:00	
6:00	
7:00	

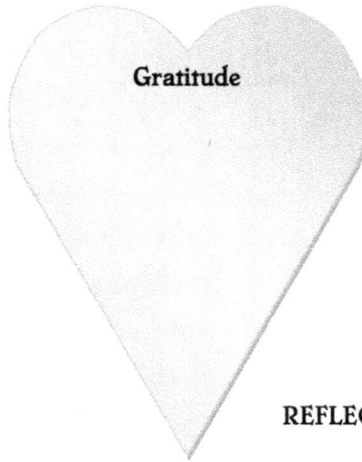

Food

Water: IIII IIII IIII

Breakfast:
_____
_____
_____

Lunch:
_____
_____
_____

Dinner:
_____
_____
_____

Snacks:
_____
_____

Notes:
_____
_____
_____

Gratitude

REFLECTION
_____
_____
_____
_____
_____
_____

DATE: _____

Morning thoughts:
_____
_____
_____
_____
_____
_____
_____

Goals & Intentions for today

1	
2	
3	
4	
5	
6	

6:00	
7:00	
8:00	
9:00	
10:00	
11:00	
12:00	
1:00	
2:00	
3:00	
4:00	
5:00	
6:00	
7:00	

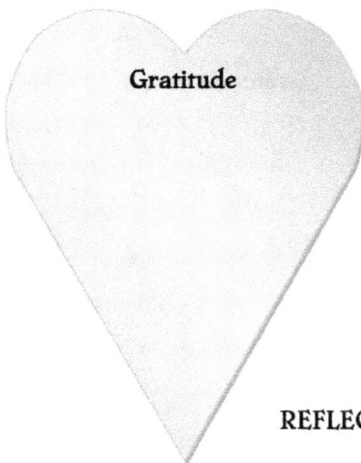

Food

Water: IIII IIII IIII

Breakfast:
_____
_____
_____

Lunch:
_____
_____
_____

Dinner:
_____
_____
_____

Snacks:
_____
_____
_____

Notes:
_____
_____
_____

Gratitude

REFLECTION
_____
_____
_____
_____
_____
_____

DATE: _____

Morning thoughts:
_____
_____
_____
_____
_____
_____
_____

Goals & Intentions for today

1
2
3
4
5
6

6:00	
7:00	
8:00	
9:00	
10:00	
11:00	
12:00	
1:00	
2:00	
3:00	
4:00	
5:00	
6:00	
7:00	

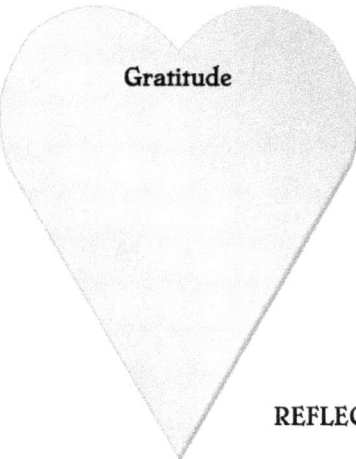

Food

Water: IIII IIII IIII

Breakfast:
_____
_____
_____

Lunch:
_____
_____
_____

Dinner:
_____
_____
_____

Snacks:
_____
_____
_____

Notes:
_____
_____
_____

Gratitude

REFLECTION
_____
_____
_____
_____
_____
_____

DATE: _____

Morning thoughts:
_____
_____
_____
_____
_____
_____
_____

Goals & Intentions for today

1	
2	
3	
4	
5	
6	

6:00	
7:00	
8:00	
9:00	
10:00	
11:00	
12:00	
1:00	
2:00	
3:00	
4:00	
5:00	
6:00	
7:00	

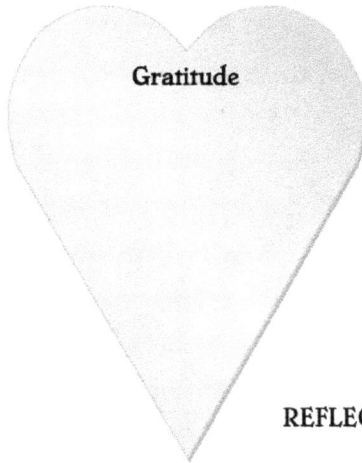

Gratitude

Food

Water: IIII IIII IIII

Breakfast:
_____
_____
_____

Lunch:
_____
_____
_____

Dinner:
_____
_____
_____

Snacks:
_____
_____

Notes:
_____
_____
_____

REFLECTION
_____
_____
_____
_____
_____
_____

155

DATE: _____

Morning thoughts:
_____
_____
_____
_____
_____
_____
_____

Goals & Intentions for today

1
2
3
4
5
6

6:00	
7:00	
8:00	
9:00	
10:00	
11:00	
12:00	
1:00	
2:00	
3:00	
4:00	
5:00	
6:00	
7:00	

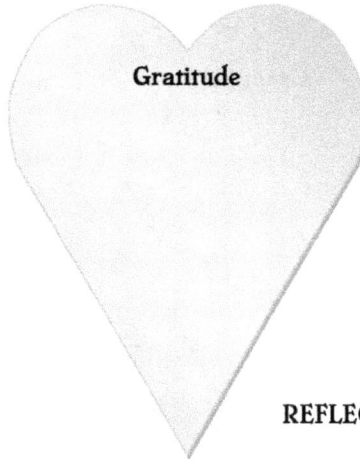

Food

Water: IIII IIII IIII

Breakfast:
_____
_____
_____

Lunch:
_____
_____
_____

Dinner:
_____
_____
_____

Snacks:
_____
_____
_____

Notes:
_____
_____
_____

Gratitude

REFLECTION

_____
_____
_____
_____
_____
_____

Journal & Schedule

Morning thoughts:
_____
_____
_____
_____
_____
_____
_____

Goals & Intentions for today

1
2
3
4
5
6

6:00	
7:00	
8:00	
9:00	
10:00	
11:00	
12:00	
1:00	
2:00	
3:00	
4:00	
5:00	
6:00	
7:00	

Food

Water: IIII IIII IIII

Breakfast:
_____
_____

Lunch:
_____
_____
_____

Dinner:
_____
_____
_____

Snacks:
_____
_____

Notes:
_____
_____
_____

Gratitude

REFLECTION
_____
_____
_____
_____
_____
_____

Journal & Schedule

Morning thoughts:
_____
_____
_____
_____
_____
_____
_____

Goals & Intentions for today

1
2
3
4
5
6

6:00	
7:00	
8:00	
9:00	
10:00	
11:00	
12:00	
1:00	
2:00	
3:00	
4:00	
5:00	
6:00	
7:00	

Food

Water: IIII IIII IIII

Breakfast:
_____
_____
_____

Lunch:
_____
_____
_____

Dinner:
_____
_____
_____

Snacks:
_____
_____
_____

Notes:
_____
_____
_____

Gratitude

REFLECTION
_____
_____
_____
_____
_____
_____

DATE: _____

Morning thoughts:

_____
_____
_____
_____
_____
_____
_____

Goals & Intentions for today

1
2
3
4
5
6

6:00	
7:00	
8:00	
9:00	
10:00	
11:00	
12:00	
1:00	
2:00	
3:00	
4:00	
5:00	
6:00	
7:00	

Food

Water: IIII IIII IIII

Breakfast:
_____
_____
_____

Lunch:
_____
_____
_____

Dinner:
_____
_____
_____

Snacks:
_____
_____

Notes:
_____
_____
_____

Gratitude

REFLECTION

_____
_____
_____
_____
_____
_____

Journal & Schedule

Morning thoughts:
_____
_____
_____
_____
_____
_____
_____

Food

Water: IIII IIII IIII

Breakfast:
_____
_____
_____

Lunch:
_____
_____
_____
_____

Dinner:
_____
_____
_____

Goals & Intentions for today

1
2
3
4
5
6

Snacks:
_____
_____
_____

Notes:
_____
_____
_____

6:00	
7:00	
8:00	
9:00	
10:00	
11:00	
12:00	
1:00	
2:00	
3:00	
4:00	
5:00	
6:00	
7:00	

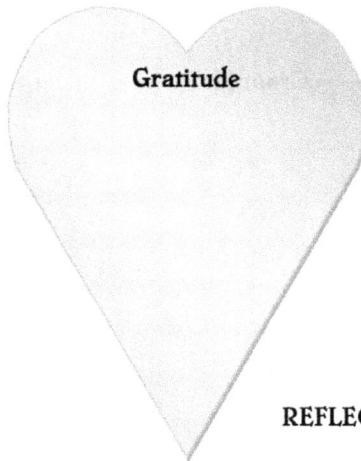

Gratitude

REFLECTION
_____
_____
_____
_____
_____
_____

DATE: _____

Morning thoughts:

_____
_____
_____
_____
_____
_____
_____

Goals & Intentions for today

1
2
3
4
5
6

6:00	
7:00	
8:00	
9:00	
10:00	
11:00	
12:00	
1:00	
2:00	
3:00	
4:00	
5:00	
6:00	
7:00	

Food

Water: IIII IIII IIII

Breakfast:
_____
_____
_____

Lunch:
_____
_____
_____

Dinner:
_____
_____
_____

Snacks:
_____
_____
_____

Notes:
_____
_____
_____

Gratitude

REFLECTION

_____
_____
_____
_____
_____
_____

Eat Vegetables First

I always think of Dr. Seuss's <u>Green Eggs and Ham</u> when I am sharing the benefits of vegetables with clients and friends. There is often so much resistance. Can't you just see it? "Could you, would you?" and the famous reply..."But I do not like them, ..."

On my personal journey, the most difficult emotional shift I needed to make around food was to move meat from the center of my plate and replace it with amazing, nutrient dense vegetables. It was difficult only because of the mindset I'd had my entire life. When it came to considering what to make for dinner, I always started with the meat. My thoughts went something like, "What am I going to make for dinner? Well, chicken and potatoes and green beans." I needed to shift this habit to be, "What am I going to make for dinner? Roots and shoots with a side of quinoa, topped with a small slice of chicken breast." You see, the meat became the optional side. It felt difficult only because of the thought pattern. Once I made the shift in my mind, the rest was easy.

--

We are just beginning to understand the role vegetables can play in our wellbeing. Nutrition is a young, complex, and ever evolving science. What we do know is that plant foods offer a diverse and deep well of nutrition that supports our body in creating energy, fighting off cancer, preventing early aging, and aiding our digestive tract. Vegetables also help us to have clear skin, sleep better, and seem to prevent a myriad of diseases. Every vegetable offers something slightly different, but the nutrients in each plant work together synergistically in a way we cannot yet recreate in a lab. What does this mean? **There is really no substitute for the real thing.**

As an example, a single cup of spinach holds 888.5 mcg (micrograms) of Vitamin K, 14742.0 IU of Vitamin A, 1.7 mg of Manganese, and 262.4 mcg of Folate. It also contains amazing amounts of Magnesium, Iron, Vitamin C, Riboflavin, Calcium, (where do you think elephants get their calcium from anyway?), Potassium, B6, Tryptophan, Fiber, Copper, B1, Protein, Phosphorus, Zinc, Vitamin E, Omega 3 Fatty Acids, Niacin, Selium, Beta-Cerotene, Lutein and Zeaxanthin. (Mateljan, 2007)

--

Adding vegetables to your diet can make a huge impact on how you feel and your ability to reach your health and wellness goals. If you would like to focus on nutrient density, the ANDI food scoring guide will help you to choose foods with an amazing nutrient power pack. The trick here is diversity. Try mixing up your vegetables and changing up how you prepare them. In the beginning, you might feel resistant, the flavors and textures might be different than what you are used to, but by sticking with it, you and your taste buds will adapt. Whole, natural, foods have flavors that vary as widely as their colors – sometimes it's in the preparation and sometimes it's in the season and growing location. Refer to the recipe section in the back of this workbook to find a few recipes to play with, or visit the recipe sections on my websites to get even more ideas.

Here is the link to the ANDI guide: http://bit.ly/1m1VGNa

Try this exercise:

Adding vegetables to your plate at every meal can be incredibly impactful. This will be a trial to identify what it feels like to have them more often and in greater amounts. As you work through the vegetables, if after a few tries you absolutely do not like a certain one, don't force yourself to eat it. We don't have to like all foods and by pushing ourselves to eat foods we dislike, we are trying to create an unsustainable habit. (I know I can't stick with eating things I don't like for very long so it's okay if you can't either.)

Begin by visiting the ANDI food scoring guide (see the link on the previous page) and choose a vegetable or two that you'd like to add to your plate over the next two weeks.

<u>Take Action & Schedule It!</u>

1. What food(s) did you choose?

2. Where will you get it?

3. When will you get it?

4. How will you prepare it?

5. How many times will you have it?

Write your plans for your meals and track your food in the journal pages of this workbook.

At the end of 14 days, come back and answer these questions:

1. What did you try?

2. How did you prepare it?

3. What was your favorite way of having it?

4. How often did you eat it?

5. How do you feel?

P.S. Try adding the vegetables you don't like to one of the smoothie recipes from the recipe section. Start with a little bit, then slowly increase the amount you add. This helps your palette to adjust to the new flavors and reminds your body what true nutrition is. Over time, you just might like it!

DATE: _____

Morning thoughts:
_____
_____
_____
_____
_____
_____
_____

Food

Water: IIII IIII IIII

Breakfast:
_____
_____

Lunch:
_____
_____
_____

Dinner:
_____
_____

Snacks:
_____
_____

Notes:
_____
_____
_____

Goals & Intentions for today

1

2

3

4

5

6

6:00	
7:00	
8:00	
9:00	
10:00	
11:00	
12:00	
1:00	
2:00	
3:00	
4:00	
5:00	
6:00	
7:00	

Gratitude

REFLECTION
_____
_____
_____
_____
_____

DATE: _____

Morning thoughts:
_____
_____
_____
_____
_____
_____
_____

Goals & Intentions for today

1	
2	
3	
4	
5	
6	

6:00	
7:00	
8:00	
9:00	
10:00	
11:00	
12:00	
1:00	
2:00	
3:00	
4:00	
5:00	
6:00	
7:00	

Food

Water: IIII IIII IIII

Breakfast:
_____
_____

Lunch:
_____
_____
_____

Dinner:
_____
_____
_____

Snacks:
_____
_____

Notes:
_____
_____
_____

Gratitude

REFLECTION
_____
_____
_____
_____
_____
_____

165

DATE: _____

Morning thoughts:
_____
_____
_____
_____
_____
_____
_____

Goals & Intentions for today

1	
2	
3	
4	
5	
6	

6:00	
7:00	
8:00	
9:00	
10:00	
11:00	
12:00	
1:00	
2:00	
3:00	
4:00	
5:00	
6:00	
7:00	

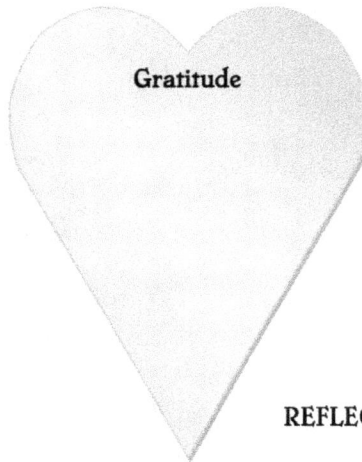

Food

Water: IIII IIII IIII

Breakfast:
_____
_____
_____

Lunch:
_____
_____
_____

Dinner:
_____
_____
_____

Snacks:
_____
_____

Notes:
_____
_____
_____

Gratitude

REFLECTION

_____
_____
_____
_____
_____
_____

DATE: _____

Morning thoughts:
_____
_____
_____
_____
_____
_____
_____

Food

Water: IIII IIII IIII

Breakfast:
_____
_____
_____

Goals & Intentions for today

1	
2	
3	
4	
5	
6	

Lunch:
_____
_____
_____

Dinner:
_____
_____
_____

Snacks:
_____
_____

6:00	
7:00	
8:00	
9:00	
10:00	
11:00	
12:00	
1:00	
2:00	
3:00	
4:00	
5:00	
6:00	
7:00	

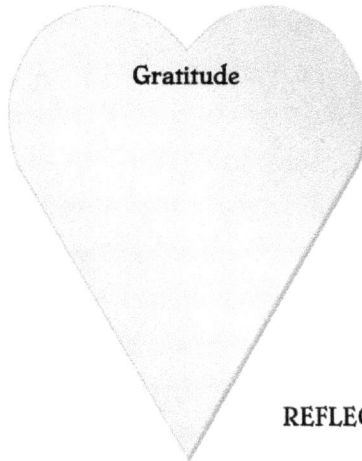

Gratitude

Notes:
_____
_____
_____
_____

REFLECTION

_____
_____
_____
_____
_____
_____

DATE: _____

Morning thoughts:
_____
_____
_____
_____
_____
_____
_____

Goals & Intentions for today

1	
2	
3	
4	
5	
6	

6:00	
7:00	
8:00	
9:00	
10:00	
11:00	
12:00	
1:00	
2:00	
3:00	
4:00	
5:00	
6:00	
7:00	

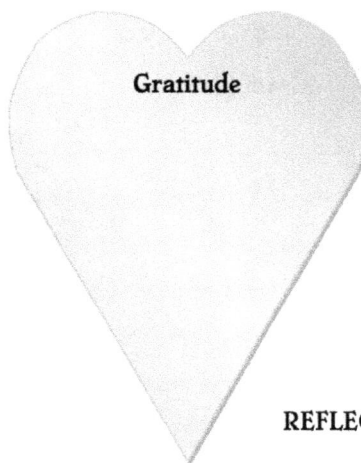

Food

Water: IIII IIII IIII

Breakfast:
_____
_____
_____

Lunch:
_____
_____
_____

Dinner:
_____
_____
_____

Snacks:
_____
_____

Notes:
_____
_____
_____

Gratitude

REFLECTION
_____
_____
_____
_____
_____
_____

DATE: _____

Morning thoughts:
_____
_____
_____
_____
_____
_____
_____

Food

Water: IIII IIII IIII

Breakfast:
_____
_____
_____

Goals & Intentions for today

1
2
3
4
5
6

Lunch:
_____
_____
_____

Dinner:
_____
_____
_____

Snacks:
_____
_____

6:00	
7:00	
8:00	
9:00	
10:00	
11:00	
12:00	
1:00	
2:00	
3:00	
4:00	
5:00	
6:00	
7:00	

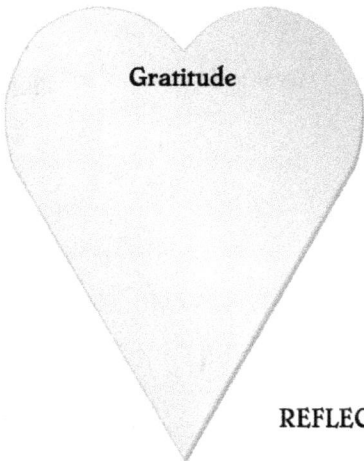

Gratitude

Notes:
_____
_____
_____

REFLECTION
_____
_____
_____
_____
_____
_____

DATE: _____

Morning thoughts:
_____
_____
_____
_____
_____
_____
_____

Food

Water: IIII IIII IIII

Breakfast:
_____
_____
_____

Goals & Intentions for today

1	
2	
3	
4	
5	
6	

Lunch:
_____
_____
_____

Dinner:
_____
_____
_____

Snacks:
_____
_____

6:00	
7:00	
8:00	
9:00	
10:00	
11:00	
12:00	
1:00	
2:00	
3:00	
4:00	
5:00	
6:00	
7:00	

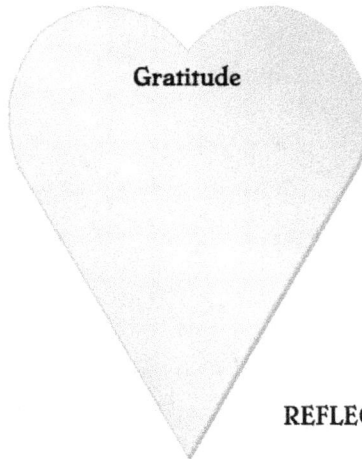

Notes:
_____
_____
_____

Gratitude

REFLECTION

_____
_____
_____
_____
_____
_____

DATE: _____

Journal & Schedule

Morning thoughts:

_____
_____
_____
_____
_____
_____

Goals & Intentions for today

1
2
3
4
5
6

6:00	
7:00	
8:00	
9:00	
10:00	
11:00	
12:00	
1:00	
2:00	
3:00	
4:00	
5:00	
6:00	
7:00	

Food

Water: IIII IIII IIII

Breakfast:
_____
_____
_____

Lunch:
_____
_____
_____

Dinner:
_____
_____
_____

Snacks:
_____
_____
_____

Notes:
_____
_____
_____
_____

Gratitude

REFLECTION

_____
_____
_____
_____
_____

DATE: _____

Morning thoughts:
_____
_____
_____
_____
_____
_____
_____

Food

Water: IIII IIII IIII

Breakfast:
_____
_____
_____

Goals & Intentions for today

1	
2	
3	
4	
5	
6	

Lunch:
_____
_____
_____

Dinner:
_____
_____
_____

Snacks:
_____
_____

Notes:
_____
_____
_____
_____

6:00	
7:00	
8:00	
9:00	
10:00	
11:00	
12:00	
1:00	
2:00	
3:00	
4:00	
5:00	
6:00	
7:00	

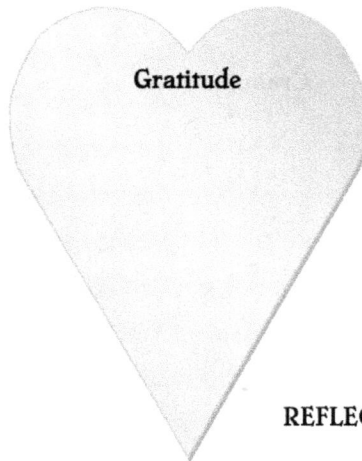

Gratitude

REFLECTION

_____
_____
_____
_____
_____
_____

DATE: _____

Journal & Schedule

Morning thoughts:
_____
_____
_____
_____
_____
_____
_____

Goals & Intentions for today

1

2

3

4

5

6

6:00	
7:00	
8:00	
9:00	
10:00	
11:00	
12:00	
1:00	
2:00	
3:00	
4:00	
5:00	
6:00	
7:00	

Gratitude

Food

Water: IIII IIII IIII

Breakfast:
_____
_____
_____

Lunch:
_____
_____
_____

Dinner:
_____
_____
_____

Snacks:
_____
_____

Notes:
_____
_____
_____

REFLECTION
_____
_____
_____
_____
_____
_____

DATE: _____

Morning thoughts:
_____
_____
_____
_____
_____
_____
_____

Goals & Intentions for today

1	
2	
3	
4	
5	
6	

6:00	
7:00	
8:00	
9:00	
10:00	
11:00	
12:00	
1:00	
2:00	
3:00	
4:00	
5:00	
6:00	
7:00	

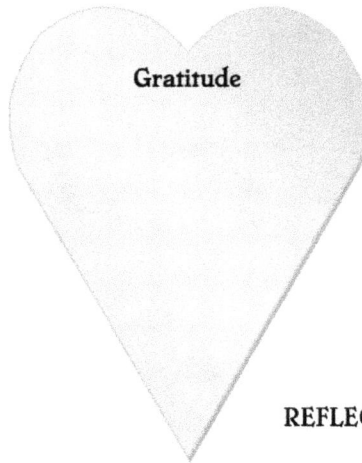

Food

Water: IIII IIII IIII

Breakfast:
_____
_____
_____

Lunch:
_____
_____
_____

Dinner:
_____
_____
_____

Snacks:
_____
_____

Notes:
_____
_____
_____

Gratitude

REFLECTION
_____
_____
_____
_____
_____
_____

DATE: _____

Morning thoughts:
_____
_____
_____
_____
_____
_____
_____

Goals & Intentions for today

1	
2	
3	
4	
5	
6	

6:00	
7:00	
8:00	
9:00	
10:00	
11:00	
12:00	
1:00	
2:00	
3:00	
4:00	
5:00	
6:00	
7:00	

Food

Water: IIII IIII IIII

Breakfast:
_____
_____
_____

Lunch:
_____
_____
_____

Dinner:
_____
_____
_____

Snacks:
_____
_____

Notes:
_____
_____
_____

Gratitude

REFLECTION

_____
_____
_____
_____
_____
_____

DATE: _____

Morning thoughts:
_____
_____
_____
_____
_____
_____
_____

Food

Water: IIII IIII IIII

Breakfast:
_____
_____
_____

Lunch:
_____
_____
_____

Goals & Intentions for today

1
2
3
4
5
6

Dinner:
_____
_____
_____

Snacks:
_____
_____

6:00	
7:00	
8:00	
9:00	
10:00	
11:00	
12:00	
1:00	
2:00	
3:00	
4:00	
5:00	
6:00	
7:00	

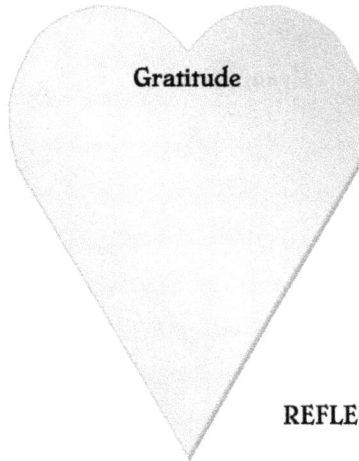

Gratitude

Notes:
_____
_____
_____
_____

REFLECTION
_____
_____
_____
_____
_____
_____

Journal & Schedule

Morning thoughts:
_____
_____
_____
_____
_____
_____
_____

Goals & Intentions for today

1
2
3
4
5
6

6:00	
7:00	
8:00	
9:00	
10:00	
11:00	
12:00	
1:00	
2:00	
3:00	
4:00	
5:00	
6:00	
7:00	

Gratitude

Food

Water: IIII IIII IIII

Breakfast:
_____
_____
_____

Lunch:
_____
_____
_____

Dinner:
_____
_____
_____

Snacks:
_____
_____

Notes:
_____
_____
_____

REFLECTION
_____
_____
_____
_____
_____

Eat Fruits Alone

I've always enjoyed eating fruit. Growing up, I don't recall having it accessible often, but it could just be because we didn't really seek it out either. As I raised my daughter, I loved to keep green seedless grapes and bananas around. The sweetest, and most alluring. They never lasted long.

Now we have fruit in our house all of the time. It feels a lot more natural to reach for an apple than a bag of chips.

--

Like vegetables, fruits offer a variety of nutrients which are diversified by freshness, plant species, and the location they are grown.

We are familiar with many healthy nutrients that fruit will deliver – for instance, we know that we'll get a load of Vitamin C when we snack on an orange, and we know that those tasty bananas are filled with Potassium. Like vegetables, there's much more to the health benefits of including fruit in your diet than these commonly known nutrients. Along with being rich in Potassium, bananas are a great source of B6, Vitamin C, Fiber, and Manganese. They also have the Carotenoids Alpha-Carotene, Beta-Carotene, and Lutein & Zeaxanthin.

Fruit digests quickly and the energy and nutrients from fruit are quickly available for the body. When fruit is eaten with more complex foods like starchy vegetables, legumes, or meat it may begin to ferment in the digestive tract. This may cause bloating and gastric discomfort.

Consider experimenting with eating fruit alone, or at least an hour before or after you eat anything else.

--

Fruit tastes absolutely amazing purchased and eaten when it is in season.

In the spring try apricots, bitter melons, limes, strawberries, honeydew, oranges, and jack fruit.

In summer look for cantaloupe, grapes, boysenberries, blueberries, blackberries, and grapefruit.

For the fall seek out Asian pear, cranberries, crab apples, huckleberries, and passion fruit.

In the winter months you can find clementines, dates, kiwi fruit, pomegranates, and tangerines.

Tips to increase fruit intake:

- ∞ Make fruit smoothies
- ∞ Replace sugary snacks with fruit
- ∞ Instead of your traditional dessert, find a dessert that includes fruit

Try this exercise:

Begin by identifying what fruits you have on hand. List them below.

Next, choose one or two fruits that you would like to add over the next two weeks.

These are:

Take Action & Schedule It!

What will you try?

When will you try it?

Where will you get it?

How will you prepare it?

Be sure to track the fruit you try in your journal portions of this workbook.

After two weeks answer these questions:

What did you notice about adding fruits to your plate over the past two weeks?

What would you like to try next?

Celebrate your success! (Perhaps with a fruit smoothie?)

DATE: _____

Morning thoughts:
_____
_____
_____
_____
_____
_____
_____

Food

Water: IIII IIII IIII

Breakfast:
_____
_____

Lunch:
_____
_____
_____

Dinner:
_____
_____
_____

Snacks:
_____
_____

Notes:
_____
_____
_____

Goals & Intentions for today

1
2
3
4
5
6

6:00	
7:00	
8:00	
9:00	
10:00	
11:00	
12:00	
1:00	
2:00	
3:00	
4:00	
5:00	
6:00	
7:00	

Gratitude

REFLECTION
_____
_____
_____
_____
_____
_____

Journal & Schedule

Morning thoughts:

_____
_____
_____
_____
_____
_____
_____

Food

Water: IIII IIII IIII

Breakfast:
_____
_____
_____

Lunch:
_____
_____
_____

Dinner:
_____
_____
_____

Snacks:
_____
_____

Notes:
_____
_____
_____

Goals & Intentions for today

1	
2	
3	
4	
5	
6	

6:00	
7:00	
8:00	
9:00	
10:00	
11:00	
12:00	
1:00	
2:00	
3:00	
4:00	
5:00	
6:00	
7:00	

Gratitude

REFLECTION

_____
_____
_____
_____
_____
_____

DATE: _____

Morning thoughts:
_____
_____
_____
_____
_____
_____
_____

Food

Water: IIII IIII IIII

Breakfast:
_____
_____
_____

Goals & Intentions for today

1
2
3
4
5
6

Lunch:
_____
_____
_____

Dinner:
_____
_____
_____

6:00	
7:00	
8:00	
9:00	
10:00	
11:00	
12:00	
1:00	
2:00	
3:00	
4:00	
5:00	
6:00	
7:00	

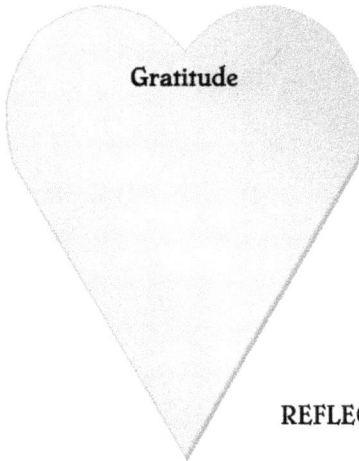

Snacks:
_____
_____

Notes:
_____
_____
_____
_____

Gratitude

REFLECTION
_____
_____
_____
_____
_____

DATE: _____

Morning thoughts:
_____
_____
_____
_____
_____
_____
_____

Goals & Intentions for today

1
2
3
4
5
6

6:00	
7:00	
8:00	
9:00	
10:00	
11:00	
12:00	
1:00	
2:00	
3:00	
4:00	
5:00	
6:00	
7:00	

Food

Water: IIII IIII IIII

Breakfast:
_____
_____
_____

Lunch:
_____
_____
_____

Dinner:
_____
_____
_____

Snacks:
_____
_____

Notes:
_____
_____
_____

Gratitude

REFLECTION
_____
_____
_____
_____
_____
_____

DATE: _____

Morning thoughts:

_____
_____
_____
_____
_____
_____
_____

Food

Water: IIII IIII IIII

Breakfast:

_____
_____
_____

Goals & Intentions for today

1	
2	
3	
4	
5	
6	

Lunch:

_____
_____
_____

Dinner:

_____
_____
_____

Snacks:

_____
_____

6:00	
7:00	
8:00	
9:00	
10:00	
11:00	
12:00	
1:00	
2:00	
3:00	
4:00	
5:00	
6:00	
7:00	

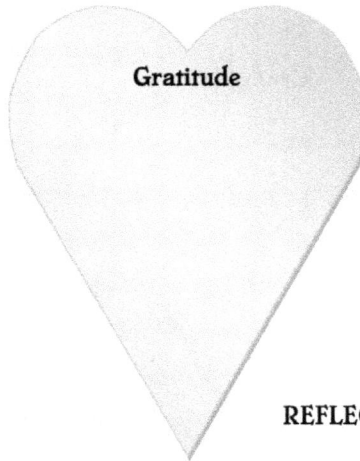

Gratitude

Notes:

_____
_____
_____

REFLECTION

_____
_____
_____
_____
_____
_____

DATE: _____

Morning thoughts:
_____
_____
_____
_____
_____
_____
_____

Food

Water: IIII IIII IIII

Breakfast:
_____
_____

Goals & Intentions for today

1
2
3
4
5
6

Lunch:
_____
_____
_____

Dinner:
_____
_____
_____

Snacks:
_____

6:00	
7:00	
8:00	
9:00	
10:00	
11:00	
12:00	
1:00	
2:00	
3:00	
4:00	
5:00	
6:00	
7:00	

Gratitude

Notes:
_____
_____
_____
_____

REFLECTION
_____
_____
_____
_____
_____
_____

DATE: _____

Morning thoughts:
_____
_____
_____
_____
_____
_____
_____

Goals & Intentions for today

1	
2	
3	
4	
5	
6	

6:00	
7:00	
8:00	
9:00	
10:00	
11:00	
12:00	
1:00	
2:00	
3:00	
4:00	
5:00	
6:00	
7:00	

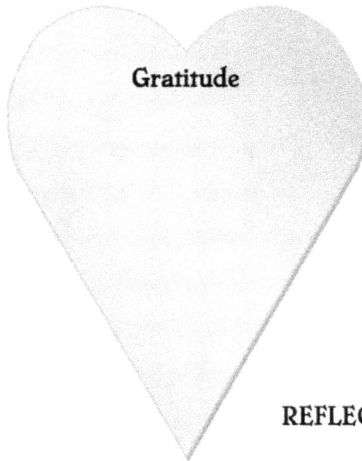

Food

Water: IIII IIII IIII

Breakfast:
_____
_____
_____

Lunch:
_____
_____
_____

Dinner:
_____
_____

Snacks:
_____
_____

Notes:
_____
_____
_____

Gratitude

REFLECTION
_____
_____
_____
_____
_____
_____

DATE: _____

Morning thoughts:
_____
_____
_____
_____
_____
_____
_____

Food

Water: IIII IIII IIII

Breakfast:
_____
_____
_____

Goals & Intentions for today

1	
2	
3	
4	
5	
6	

Lunch:
_____
_____
_____

Dinner:
_____
_____
_____

Snacks:
_____

6:00	
7:00	
8:00	
9:00	
10:00	
11:00	
12:00	
1:00	
2:00	
3:00	
4:00	
5:00	
6:00	
7:00	

Notes:
_____
_____
_____
_____

Gratitude

REFLECTION
_____
_____
_____
_____
_____
_____

Journal & Schedule

Morning thoughts:

_____
_____
_____
_____
_____
_____
_____

Goals & Intentions for today

1
2
3
4
5
6

6:00	
7:00	
8:00	
9:00	
10:00	
11:00	
12:00	
1:00	
2:00	
3:00	
4:00	
5:00	
6:00	
7:00	

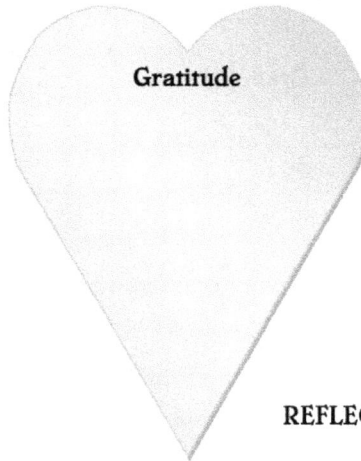

Food

Water: IIII IIII IIII

Breakfast:

_____
_____
_____

Lunch:

_____
_____
_____

Dinner:

_____
_____
_____

Snacks:

_____
_____
_____

Notes:

_____
_____
_____

Gratitude

REFLECTION

_____
_____
_____
_____
_____
_____

DATE: _____

Morning thoughts:
_____
_____
_____
_____
_____
_____
_____

Goals & Intentions for today

1
2
3
4
5
6

6:00	
7:00	
8:00	
9:00	
10:00	
11:00	
12:00	
1:00	
2:00	
3:00	
4:00	
5:00	
6:00	
7:00	

Gratitude

REFLECTION
_____
_____
_____
_____
_____
_____

Food

Water: IIII IIII IIII
Breakfast:
_____
_____

Lunch:
_____
_____
_____

Dinner:
_____
_____
_____

Snacks:
_____
_____

Notes:
_____
_____
_____

DATE: _____

Morning thoughts:
_____
_____
_____
_____
_____
_____
_____

Food

Water: IIII IIII IIII

Breakfast:
_____
_____

Goals & Intentions for today

1
2
3
4
5
6

Lunch:
_____
_____
_____

Dinner:
_____
_____
_____

Snacks:
_____
_____

6:00	
7:00	
8:00	
9:00	
10:00	
11:00	
12:00	
1:00	
2:00	
3:00	
4:00	
5:00	
6:00	
7:00	

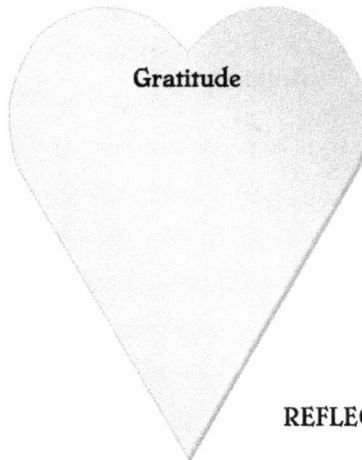

Notes:
_____
_____
_____

Gratitude

REFLECTION

_____
_____
_____
_____
_____
_____

DATE: _____

Morning thoughts:
_____
_____
_____
_____
_____
_____
_____

Food

Water: IIII IIII IIII

Breakfast:
_____
_____
_____

Goals & Intentions for today

1	
2	
3	
4	
5	
6	

Lunch:
_____
_____
_____

Dinner:
_____
_____
_____

Snacks:
_____
_____
_____

Notes:
_____
_____
_____

6:00	
7:00	
8:00	
9:00	
10:00	
11:00	
12:00	
1:00	
2:00	
3:00	
4:00	
5:00	
6:00	
7:00	

Gratitude

REFLECTION
_____
_____
_____
_____
_____
_____

Journal & Schedule

Morning thoughts:
_____
_____
_____
_____
_____
_____
_____

Goals & Intentions for today

1
2
3
4
5
6

6:00	
7:00	
8:00	
9:00	
10:00	
11:00	
12:00	
1:00	
2:00	
3:00	
4:00	
5:00	
6:00	
7:00	

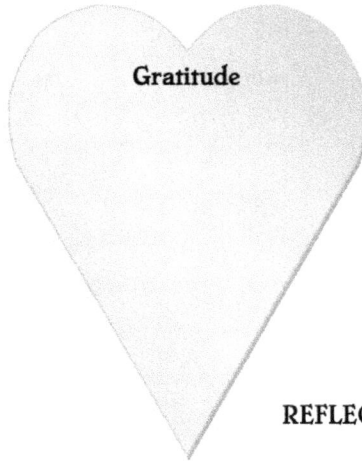

Gratitude

Food

Water: IIII IIII IIII

Breakfast:
_____
_____
_____

Lunch:
_____
_____
_____

Dinner:
_____
_____
_____

Snacks:
_____
_____

Notes:
_____
_____
_____

REFLECTION
_____
_____
_____
_____
_____
_____

DATE: _____

Morning thoughts:

_____
_____
_____
_____
_____
_____
_____

Food

Water: IIII IIII IIII

Breakfast:
_____
_____
_____

Goals & Intentions for today

1

2

3

4

5

6

Lunch:
_____
_____
_____

Dinner:
_____
_____
_____

Snacks:
_____
_____

Notes:
_____
_____
_____
_____
_____

6:00	
7:00	
8:00	
9:00	
10:00	
11:00	
12:00	
1:00	
2:00	
3:00	
4:00	
5:00	
6:00	
7:00	

Gratitude

REFLECTION

_____
_____
_____
_____
_____
_____

Eat Whole Grains

I had never had brown rice in my life. Those first few times, it tasted so different. Then something happened. It was as if my body received life blood for the first time. I began craving grains. Rice, quinoa, kasha, millet, oats. It didn't matter!

I needed more!

For four solid months I ate a huge helping of whole grains at every meal. Then the craving stopped.

--

Whole grains like rice, millet, kasha, quinoa, buckwheat, and oats provide a different spectrum of nutrients than vegetables.

I call these the feel good foods because they contain the B-complex vitamins. Have you ever craved carbs when you are feeling blue? Your body is pretty smart! The challenge is that most processed grain products have had these very nutrients stripped out during the refinement process; then a manmade substitute was added back in to replace part of the nutrients that were removed. A slice of bread, white or wheat, just isn't going to give you the same physical or emotional satisfaction as a ¼ cup of brown rice or steel cut oats.

Whole grains are also a great source of sustainable energy. They take a little more time for the body to break down, give you a feeling of fullness, and help you to feel more satisfied.

Cooking Guide for Whole Grains:

Always rinse your grains really well to reduce the naturally occurring phytic acid and saponins that will impart a bitter flavor and inhibit nutrient absorption. Remove any visible debris.

Some grains require soaking to help break the grain down and to further reduce the phytic acid. It's especially helpful to soak your rice. Do not soak buckwheat or it will get mushy. Before cooking millet, try toasting it quickly in a frying pan to give it a nuttier flavor. All suggested times and measurements are approximate. It's a good idea to read the package directions before beginning and to follow those directly.

Because grains take a little while to cook, it's a great idea to cook extra and use the remaining grains in more meals. To add an amazing flavor to your grains, try substituting part or all of the water with vegetable or chicken broth.

1 Cup of Grain Type	Amount of Water	Cooking Time
Quinoa	2 C.	20 minutes
Brown Rice	2 C.	50 minutes
Rolled Oats	2 C.	50 minutes
Toasted Buckwheat (Kasha)	1 C.	20 minutes
Millet	2 C.	30 minutes
Wild Rice	4 C.	60 minutes

Try this exercise:

First, identify where you are currently with whole grains by checking your cabinets. What do you already have on hand? List it here:

What would you like to try?

<u>TAKE ACTION & SCHEDULE IT!</u>

Meal planning can be a priceless tool when it comes to feeding yourself and your family well. Doing so allows you to be prepared.

Using your personal planner or calendar, select three days during the next week that you will serve whole grains. Next, find one or two recipes you'd like to try that include the grains you've chosen. Write this in your planner. Do the same for the following week. Be sure to track your new grains in the food portion of the workbook.

At the end of the two weeks, come back and answer these questions:

How did this experiment go?

What did you notice about including these foods in your diet?

How does your body feel? How did you feel during meals? After meals?

What did you enjoy about this process?

What will you do differently next time?

P.S. To save time and energy, I choose a single grain to serve at many meals every week. On Sunday, I will cook enough to use for all the meals I plan – then toss the meal portions already separated into the fridge or even better, the freezer. This saves so much time during the week and it makes eating these wonderful foods SUPER EASY!

DATE: _____

Morning thoughts:
_____
_____
_____
_____
_____
_____
_____

Food

Water: IIII IIII IIII

Breakfast:
_____
_____
_____

Lunch:
_____
_____
_____

Goals & Intentions for today

1
2
3
4
5
6

Dinner:
_____
_____
_____

Snacks:
_____
_____

6:00	
7:00	
8:00	
9:00	
10:00	
11:00	
12:00	
1:00	
2:00	
3:00	
4:00	
5:00	
6:00	
7:00	

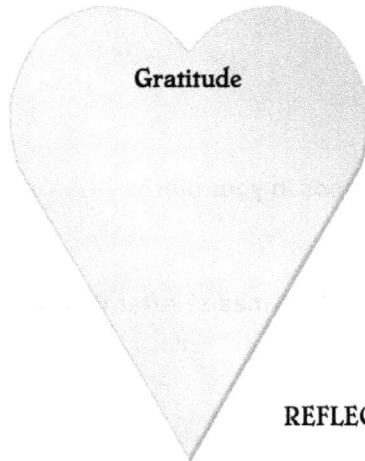

Gratitude

Notes:
_____
_____
_____
_____

REFLECTION

_____
_____
_____
_____
_____
_____

DATE: _____

Morning thoughts:
_____
_____
_____
_____
_____
_____
_____

Goals & Intentions for today

1
2
3
4
5
6

6:00	
7:00	
8:00	
9:00	
10:00	
11:00	
12:00	
1:00	
2:00	
3:00	
4:00	
5:00	
6:00	
7:00	

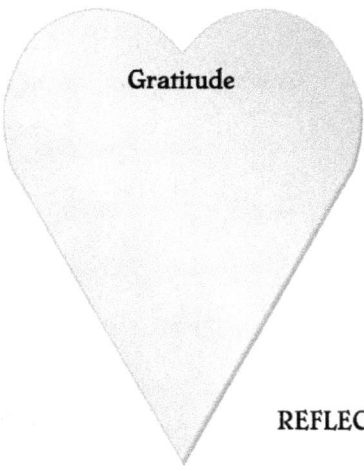

Food

Water: IIII IIII IIII

Breakfast:
_____
_____
_____

Lunch:
_____
_____
_____

Dinner:
_____
_____

Snacks:
_____
_____

Notes:
_____
_____
_____

Gratitude

REFLECTION

_____
_____
_____
_____
_____
_____

DATE: _____

Morning thoughts:
_____
_____
_____
_____
_____
_____
_____

Goals & Intentions for today

1
2
3
4
5
6

6:00	
7:00	
8:00	
9:00	
10:00	
11:00	
12:00	
1:00	
2:00	
3:00	
4:00	
5:00	
6:00	
7:00	

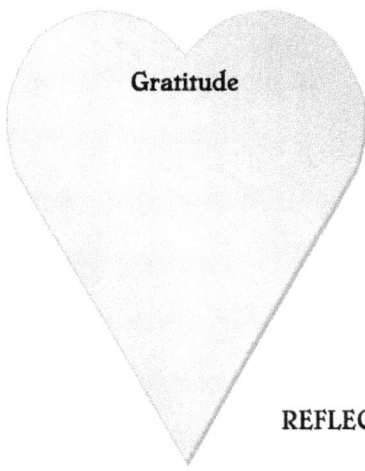

Food

Water: IIII IIII IIII

Breakfast:
_____
_____
_____

Lunch:
_____
_____
_____

Dinner:
_____
_____
_____

Snacks:
_____
_____

Notes:
_____
_____
_____
_____

Gratitude

REFLECTION
_____
_____
_____
_____
_____
_____

DATE: _____

Morning thoughts:
_____
_____
_____
_____
_____
_____
_____

Food

Water: IIII IIII IIII

Breakfast:
_____
_____
_____

Goals & Intentions for today

1	
2	
3	
4	
5	
6	

Lunch:
_____
_____
_____

Dinner:
_____
_____
_____

Snacks:
_____
_____
_____

6:00	
7:00	
8:00	
9:00	
10:00	
11:00	
12:00	
1:00	
2:00	
3:00	
4:00	
5:00	
6:00	
7:00	

Gratitude

Notes:
_____
_____
_____

REFLECTION
_____
_____
_____
_____
_____
_____

Journal & Schedule

Morning thoughts:
_____
_____
_____
_____
_____
_____
_____

Goals & Intentions for today

1
2
3
4
5
6

6:00	
7:00	
8:00	
9:00	
10:00	
11:00	
12:00	
1:00	
2:00	
3:00	
4:00	
5:00	
6:00	
7:00	

Gratitude

Food

Water: IIII IIII IIII

Breakfast:
_____
_____
_____

Lunch:
_____
_____
_____

Dinner:
_____
_____
_____

Snacks:
_____
_____
_____

Notes:
_____
_____
_____

REFLECTION
_____
_____
_____
_____
_____
_____

DATE: _____

Morning thoughts:

_____
_____
_____
_____
_____
_____
_____

Goals & Intentions for today

1
2
3
4
5
6

6:00	
7:00	
8:00	
9:00	
10:00	
11:00	
12:00	
1:00	
2:00	
3:00	
4:00	
5:00	
6:00	
7:00	

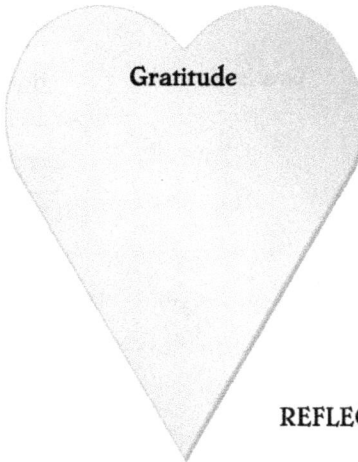

Gratitude

Food

Water: IIII IIII IIII

Breakfast:
_____
_____
_____

Lunch:
_____
_____
_____

Dinner:
_____
_____
_____

Snacks:
_____
_____

Notes:
_____
_____
_____

REFLECTION

_____
_____
_____
_____
_____
_____

Journal & Schedule

Morning thoughts:
_____
_____
_____
_____
_____
_____
_____

Goals & Intentions for today

1
2
3
4
5
6

6:00	
7:00	
8:00	
9:00	
10:00	
11:00	
12:00	
1:00	
2:00	
3:00	
4:00	
5:00	
6:00	
7:00	

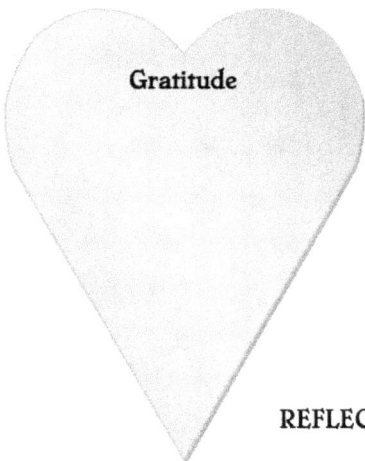

Gratitude

Food

Water: IIII IIII IIII

Breakfast:
_____
_____
_____

Lunch:
_____
_____
_____

Dinner:
_____
_____
_____

Snacks:
_____
_____

Notes:
_____
_____
_____
_____

REFLECTION

_____
_____
_____
_____
_____
_____

DATE: _____

Morning thoughts:

_____
_____
_____
_____
_____
_____
_____

Food

Water: IIII IIII IIII

Breakfast:

_____
_____
_____

Lunch:

_____
_____
_____

Dinner:

_____
_____
_____

Snacks:

_____
_____
_____

Notes:

_____
_____
_____
_____

Goals & Intentions for today

1	
2	
3	
4	
5	
6	

6:00	
7:00	
8:00	
9:00	
10:00	
11:00	
12:00	
1:00	
2:00	
3:00	
4:00	
5:00	
6:00	
7:00	

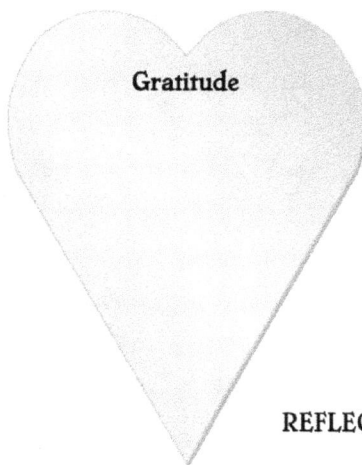

Gratitude

REFLECTION

_____
_____
_____
_____
_____
_____

Journal & Schedule

Morning thoughts:
_____
_____
_____
_____
_____
_____
_____

Goals & Intentions for today

1
2
3
4
5
6

6:00	
7:00	
8:00	
9:00	
10:00	
11:00	
12:00	
1:00	
2:00	
3:00	
4:00	
5:00	
6:00	
7:00	

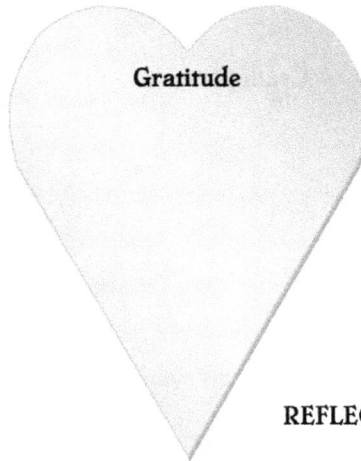

Food

Water: IIII IIII IIII

Breakfast:
_____
_____
_____

Lunch:
_____
_____
_____

Dinner:
_____
_____

Snacks:
_____
_____

Notes:
_____
_____
_____

Gratitude

REFLECTION
_____
_____
_____
_____
_____
_____

DATE: _____

Morning thoughts:

_____
_____
_____
_____
_____
_____
_____

Food

Water: IIII IIII IIII

Breakfast:
_____
_____
_____

Lunch:
_____
_____
_____

Dinner:
_____
_____
_____

Snacks:
_____
_____

Notes:
_____
_____
_____

Goals & Intentions for today

1
2
3
4
5
6

6:00	
7:00	
8:00	
9:00	
10:00	
11:00	
12:00	
1:00	
2:00	
3:00	
4:00	
5:00	
6:00	
7:00	

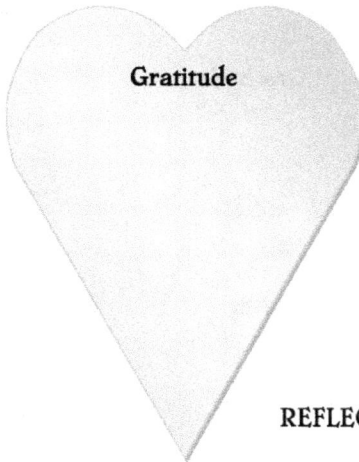

Gratitude

REFLECTION

_____
_____
_____
_____
_____
_____

DATE: _____

Morning thoughts:
_____
_____
_____
_____
_____
_____
_____

Food

Water: IIII IIII IIII

Breakfast:
_____
_____
_____

Goals & Intentions for today

1
2
3
4
5
6

Lunch:
_____
_____
_____

Dinner:
_____
_____
_____

Snacks:
_____
_____

6:00	
7:00	
8:00	
9:00	
10:00	
11:00	
12:00	
1:00	
2:00	
3:00	
4:00	
5:00	
6:00	
7:00	

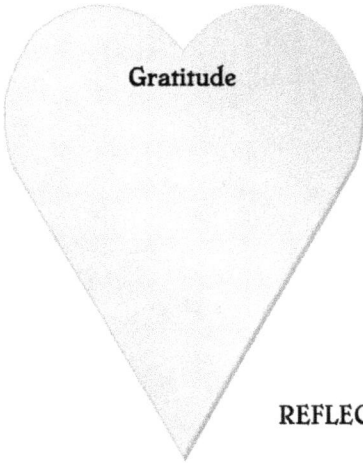

Notes:
_____
_____
_____
_____

Gratitude

REFLECTION
_____
_____
_____
_____
_____
_____

DATE: _____

Morning thoughts:
_____
_____
_____
_____
_____
_____
_____

Goals & Intentions for today

1	
2	
3	
4	
5	
6	

6:00	
7:00	
8:00	
9:00	
10:00	
11:00	
12:00	
1:00	
2:00	
3:00	
4:00	
5:00	
6:00	
7:00	

Food

Water: IIII IIII IIII

Breakfast:
_____
_____
_____

Lunch:
_____
_____
_____

Dinner:
_____
_____
_____

Snacks:
_____
_____
_____

Notes:
_____
_____
_____

Gratitude

REFLECTION
_____
_____
_____
_____
_____
_____

DATE: _____

Morning thoughts:
_____
_____
_____
_____
_____
_____
_____

Food

Water: IIII IIII IIII

Breakfast:
_____
_____
_____

Goals & Intentions for today

1

2

3

4

5

6

Lunch:
_____
_____
_____

Dinner:
_____
_____
_____

Snacks:
_____
_____

6:00	
7:00	
8:00	
9:00	
10:00	
11:00	
12:00	
1:00	
2:00	
3:00	
4:00	
5:00	
6:00	
7:00	

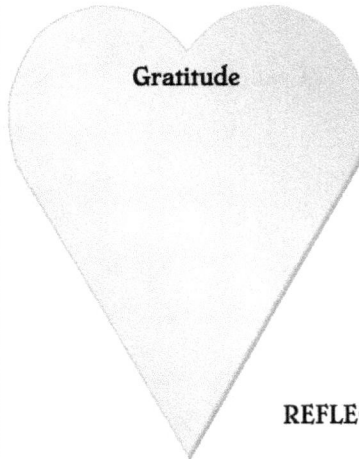

Gratitude

Notes:
_____
_____
_____
_____

REFLECTION

_____
_____
_____
_____
_____

DATE: _____

Morning thoughts:

_____
_____
_____
_____
_____
_____
_____

Food

Water: IIII IIII IIII

Breakfast:
_____
_____
_____

Goals & Intentions for today

1
2
3
4
5
6

Lunch:
_____
_____
_____

Dinner:
_____
_____
_____

Snacks:
_____
_____
_____

6:00	
7:00	
8:00	
9:00	
10:00	
11:00	
12:00	
1:00	
2:00	
3:00	
4:00	
5:00	
6:00	
7:00	

Gratitude

Notes:
_____
_____
_____

REFLECTION

_____
_____
_____
_____
_____
_____

Eat Seeds

When I found out flax seeds would add Omega 3's to our diet, I was putting them in everything. We were having flax pancakes, flax in our smoothies and flax on our yogurt.

I learned how to make flax crackers in our dehydrator and mix them into homemade granolas. Then chia seeds came along. ....

--

Seeds are an easy and tasteful way to add variety and depth to your plate. Seeds are often easier to digest than grains and all have a unique nutrient profile.

Pumpkin seeds contain Manganese, Magnesium, Phosphorus, Tryptophan, Iron, Copper, Vitamin K, Zinc, and Protein. Sesame seeds contain a large variety of Amino Acids like Arginine, Glycine, and Cystine, Vitamins like A, B Complex, D, E, Folate, and K, and Omega's 3 and 6. They are also rich in minerals like Calcium, and Potassium. Pumpkin seeds, when eaten raw also have anti-parasitic properties.

Sunflower seeds are rich in Vitamin E, Thiamin, Manganese, Magnesium, Copper, Tryptophan, Selenium, Pantothenic Acid and Folate. Because seeds are the beginning of a new life, they are a concentrated and complex source of nutrients.

--

Seeds to try and a few of their benefits (Mateljan, 2007)

- ∞ Sunflower Seeds: Promote heart health, brain health, over all optimal health
- ∞ Flax Seeds: Promote Women's breast health, digestive health
- ∞ Sesame Seeds: Promote joint and skin health, bone health, healthy sleep
- ∞ Pumpkin Seeds: Promotes men's health, joint health

For best results, store your seeds in the refrigerator. Seeds may be toasted, baked, or eaten raw.

Tips for getting in more seeds:

- ∞ Add to baked goods
- ∞ Top your salad
- ∞ Toss some in a smoothie
- ∞ Use as a snack
- ∞ Top a potato
- ∞ Use mixed in with or to replace a breading on fish or chicken

Try this exercise:

Choose one or two types of seeds to try over the next two weeks. Write them here:

Identify two or three recipes that include these. A great place to find beautiful and tasty recipes is by using a website called Pinterest. (Pinterest.com) You might also try Googling "Recipes with _____". You may also add your seeds to any of the smoothie recipes in the recipe section of this workbook.

You'll notice a variety of the recipes included already have seeds in the recipe.

How will you prepare your seeds?

Where will you get them?

When will you get them?

TAKE ACTION & SCHEDULE IT!

Log in your journal pages over the next two weeks the recipes that you intend to make that include these seeds.

After these two weeks, return to this page to answer the following:

What were your favorite seed recipes/seeds?

What did you notice about including these in your diet?

Are you feeling hungry, overly full, or satisfied after eating?

Do you want to continue adding seeds to your recipes/diet?

Which will you try next?

Journal & Schedule

Morning thoughts:
_____
_____
_____
_____
_____
_____
_____

Goals & Intentions for today

1
2
3
4
5
6

6:00	
7:00	
8:00	
9:00	
10:00	
11:00	
12:00	
1:00	
2:00	
3:00	
4:00	
5:00	
6:00	
7:00	

Food

Water: IIII IIII IIII

Breakfast:
_____
_____

Lunch:
_____
_____
_____

Dinner:
_____
_____

Snacks:
_____
_____

Notes:
_____
_____
_____

Gratitude

REFLECTION
_____
_____
_____
_____
_____
_____

DATE: _____

Morning thoughts:
_____
_____
_____
_____
_____
_____
_____

Goals & Intentions for today

1
2
3
4
5
6

6:00	
7:00	
8:00	
9:00	
10:00	
11:00	
12:00	
1:00	
2:00	
3:00	
4:00	
5:00	
6:00	
7:00	

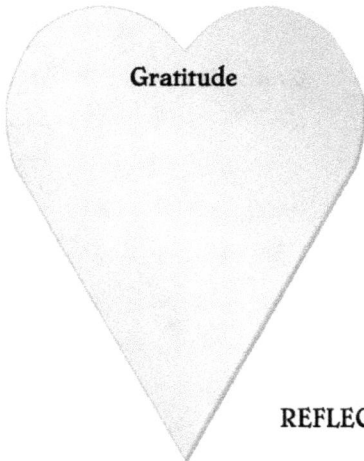

Food

Water: IIII IIII IIII

Breakfast:
_____
_____
_____

Lunch:
_____
_____
_____

Dinner:
_____
_____
_____

Snacks:
_____
_____
_____

Notes:
_____
_____
_____

Gratitude

REFLECTION
_____
_____
_____
_____
_____
_____

DATE: _____

Morning thoughts:
_____
_____
_____
_____
_____
_____
_____

Goals & Intentions for today

1

2

3

4

5

6

6:00	
7:00	
8:00	
9:00	
10:00	
11:00	
12:00	
1:00	
2:00	
3:00	
4:00	
5:00	
6:00	
7:00	

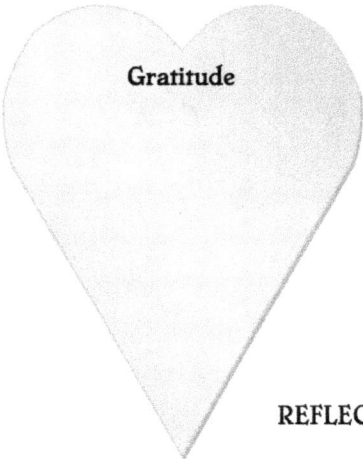

Food

Water: IIII IIII IIII

Breakfast:
_____
_____
_____

Lunch:
_____
_____
_____

Dinner:
_____
_____

Snacks:
_____
_____

Notes:
_____
_____
_____
_____

Gratitude

REFLECTION

_____
_____
_____
_____
_____
_____

DATE: _____

Morning thoughts:
_____
_____
_____
_____
_____
_____
_____

Goals & Intentions for today

1	
2	
3	
4	
5	
6	

6:00	
7:00	
8:00	
9:00	
10:00	
11:00	
12:00	
1:00	
2:00	
3:00	
4:00	
5:00	
6:00	
7:00	

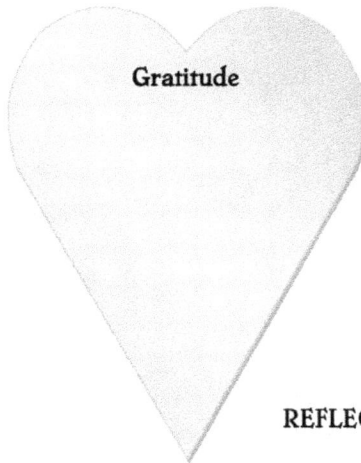

Food

Water: IIII IIII IIII

Breakfast:
_____
_____

Lunch:
_____
_____
_____

Dinner:
_____
_____

Snacks:
_____
_____

Notes:
_____
_____
_____

Gratitude

REFLECTION
_____
_____
_____
_____
_____
_____

DATE: _____

Morning thoughts:
_____
_____
_____
_____
_____
_____
_____

Food

Water: IIII IIII IIII

Breakfast:
_____
_____
_____

Goals & Intentions for today

| 1 |
| 2 |
| 3 |
| 4 |
| 5 |
| 6 |

Lunch:
_____
_____
_____

Dinner:
_____
_____
_____

Snacks:
_____
_____
_____

Notes:
_____
_____
_____

6:00	
7:00	
8:00	
9:00	
10:00	
11:00	
12:00	
1:00	
2:00	
3:00	
4:00	
5:00	
6:00	
7:00	

Gratitude

REFLECTION
_____
_____
_____
_____
_____
_____

DATE: _____

Morning thoughts:
_____
_____
_____
_____
_____
_____
_____

Goals & Intentions for today

1
2
3
4
5
6

6:00	
7:00	
8:00	
9:00	
10:00	
11:00	
12:00	
1:00	
2:00	
3:00	
4:00	
5:00	
6:00	
7:00	

Food

Water: IIII IIII IIII

Breakfast:
_____
_____
_____

Lunch:
_____
_____
_____

Dinner:
_____
_____
_____

Snacks:
_____
_____
_____

Notes:
_____
_____
_____

Gratitude

REFLECTION
_____
_____
_____
_____
_____
_____

DATE: _____

Morning thoughts:
_____
_____
_____
_____
_____
_____
_____

Goals & Intentions for today

1	
2	
3	
4	
5	
6	

6:00	
7:00	
8:00	
9:00	
10:00	
11:00	
12:00	
1:00	
2:00	
3:00	
4:00	
5:00	
6:00	
7:00	

Food

Water: IIII IIII IIII

Breakfast:
_____
_____
_____

Lunch:
_____
_____
_____

Dinner:
_____
_____
_____

Snacks:
_____
_____
_____

Notes:
_____
_____
_____

Gratitude

REFLECTION
_____
_____
_____
_____
_____
_____

Morning thoughts:

_____
_____
_____
_____
_____
_____

Food

Water: IIII IIII IIII

Breakfast:

_____
_____
_____

Lunch:

_____
_____
_____

Goals & Intentions for today

1

2

3

4

5

6

Dinner:

_____
_____
_____

Snacks:

_____
_____
_____

6:00	
7:00	
8:00	
9:00	
10:00	
11:00	
12:00	
1:00	
2:00	
3:00	
4:00	
5:00	
6:00	
7:00	

Gratitude

Notes:

_____
_____
_____

REFLECTION

_____
_____
_____
_____
_____

Journal & Schedule

Morning thoughts:
_____
_____
_____
_____
_____
_____
_____

Goals & Intentions for today

1
2
3
4
5
6

6:00	
7:00	
8:00	
9:00	
10:00	
11:00	
12:00	
1:00	
2:00	
3:00	
4:00	
5:00	
6:00	
7:00	

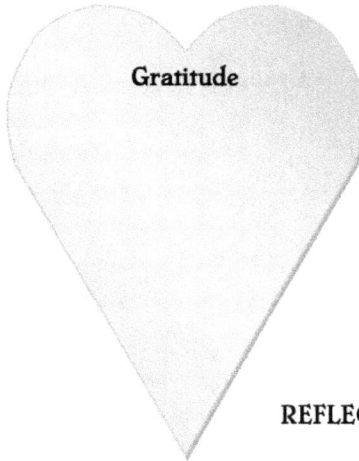

Food

Water: IIII IIII IIII

Breakfast:
_____
_____

Lunch:
_____
_____
_____

Dinner:
_____
_____
_____

Snacks:
_____
_____

Notes:
_____
_____
_____

Gratitude

REFLECTION
_____
_____
_____
_____
_____
_____

DATE: _____

Morning thoughts:
_____
_____
_____
_____
_____
_____
_____

Goals & Intentions for today

1	
2	
3	
4	
5	
6	

6:00	
7:00	
8:00	
9:00	
10:00	
11:00	
12:00	
1:00	
2:00	
3:00	
4:00	
5:00	
6:00	
7:00	

Food

Water: IIII IIII IIII

Breakfast:
_____
_____
_____

Lunch:
_____
_____
_____

Dinner:
_____
_____
_____

Snacks:
_____
_____
_____

Notes:
_____
_____
_____

Gratitude

REFLECTION
_____
_____
_____
_____
_____

DATE: _____

Morning thoughts:
_____
_____
_____
_____
_____
_____
_____

Food

Water: IIII IIII IIII

Breakfast:
_____
_____
_____

Lunch:
_____
_____
_____

Goals & Intentions for today

1

2

3

4

5

6

Dinner:
_____
_____

Snacks:
_____
_____

6:00	
7:00	
8:00	
9:00	
10:00	
11:00	
12:00	
1:00	
2:00	
3:00	
4:00	
5:00	
6:00	
7:00	

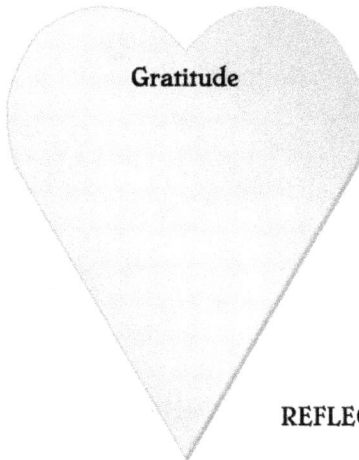

Notes:
_____
_____
_____
_____

Gratitude

REFLECTION
_____
_____
_____
_____
_____
_____

DATE: _____

Morning thoughts:
_____
_____
_____
_____
_____
_____
_____

Food

Water: IIII IIII IIII

Breakfast:
_____
_____
_____

Lunch:
_____
_____
_____

Goals & Intentions for today

1	
2	
3	
4	
5	
6	

Dinner:
_____
_____
_____

Snacks:
_____
_____

Notes:
_____
_____
_____
_____

6:00	
7:00	
8:00	
9:00	
10:00	
11:00	
12:00	
1:00	
2:00	
3:00	
4:00	
5:00	
6:00	
7:00	

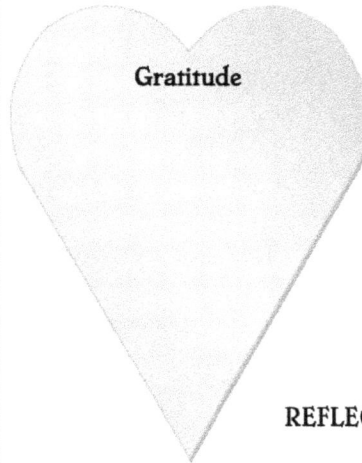

Gratitude

REFLECTION
_____
_____
_____
_____
_____

DATE: _____

Morning thoughts:
_____
_____
_____
_____
_____
_____
_____

Goals & Intentions for today

1
2
3
4
5
6

6:00	
7:00	
8:00	
9:00	
10:00	
11:00	
12:00	
1:00	
2:00	
3:00	
4:00	
5:00	
6:00	
7:00	

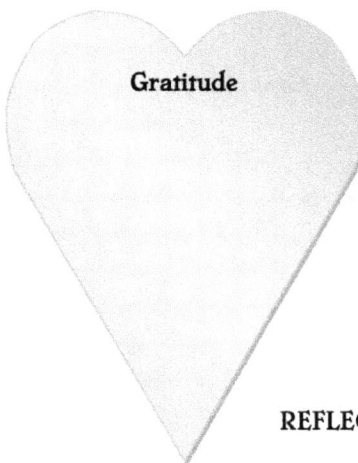

Gratitude

Food

Water: IIII IIII IIII

Breakfast:
_____
_____
_____

Lunch:
_____
_____
_____

Dinner:
_____
_____
_____

Snacks:
_____
_____
_____

Notes:
_____
_____
_____

REFLECTION

_____
_____
_____
_____
_____
_____

Journal & Schedule

Morning thoughts:
_____
_____
_____
_____
_____
_____
_____

Goals & Intentions for today

1
2
3
4
5
6

6:00	
7:00	
8:00	
9:00	
10:00	
11:00	
12:00	
1:00	
2:00	
3:00	
4:00	
5:00	
6:00	
7:00	

Food

Water: IIII IIII IIII

Breakfast:
_____
_____
_____

Lunch:
_____
_____
_____

Dinner:
_____
_____
_____

Snacks:
_____
_____

Notes:
_____
_____
_____

Gratitude

REFLECTION
_____
_____
_____
_____
_____
_____

Eat Local

For 16 years, my family and I lived on the Colorado prairie. On 35 acres, my husband "broke his back" to build our home - at night and on the weekends; a house, a barn, a wood shop, a greenhouse....which was quite extensive. It was what he amicably called his compound. Over the years, we planted and learned to grow our own food. It's a romantic idea for a city girl, but the reality is that it's very difficult work. The land was parched of both water and nutrients. The weeds grew like rabbits have litters. Every year we worked against nature - hail, rain, hot sun, drought, and wild animals. Over time, we learned how to successfully plant and grow a tree, how to grow green chilies and tomatoes that were deep in flavor and color, and to limit the mounds of zucchini.

During the last few years of our time in this place, we made the decision to get our own chickens. Following the inspiration of my husband's oldest brother, we ordered almost 80 birds – a straight run of chickens and pheasant. It was a dream come true for me, losing only one to sickness, the birds went without antibiotics, were snuggled with daily so they were friendly. We enjoyed this adventure immensely.

In the end, and in reflection, this was the greatest adventure of my life so far. I will always miss that place dearly. It was my home – the first one I'd really had in my life. In a way, it was the beginning of the foundation for my family. I raised my children there, had more furry pets than I can count, grew flowers and herbs of every name and color, and watched as time passed by. This is where I grew, strengthened, and healed my inner wounds. There is nothing like reaping what you sow. The long hot days under the sun gave way to evening gatherings filled with Earth's sweetest abundance of life giving, health granting foods. My family – husband, son, daughter, and myself; would gather around the stone fire place and roast vegetables followed by the sweetest S'mores. Life was truly full and good.

--

Do you have a vegetable garden? How about your parents? How about your grandparents? How about your Great-Grandparents? Somewhere along the way, we lost our roots – our connection to our food. We stopped growing food for ourselves. Gardens are now for hobbies instead of sustenance and we rely on big business to feed us and our children instead. How did this happen? Why?

While it's not always practical for everyone to have a garden, eating food that is grown locally can have a profound impact on your health and the environment.

The typical distance from farm to table varies from 1500 – 2500 miles and much of it is imported. This distance negatively impacts the economic wellbeing of local farms, increases opportunity for contamination and spoilage, and increases the need for artificial flavorings, preservatives, and colors. This distance also greatly impacts the flavor and nutrient bio-availability of the food. Fruits and vegetables are at their peak nutrient availability at the time of picking. As the live enzymes die off, the food loses its powerful punch. Let's just say kale and kiwi from 1,000 miles away two weeks ago is going to have a completely different health and environmental impact than kale and kiwi from your neighborhood farm, or better, from your backyard.

There are certainly great options to choose from as you make a shift from buying food from the other side of the world, to foods that are grown in your state or local community. One option is to grow your own; another is to visit a farmer's market in your area. There are still other options. A way to find out what options are available to you is to visit localharvest.org. Here you'll find a list of farmer's market and CSA (Community

Supported Agriculture) options based on your location. There are also helpful apps available for your smart devices, such as Locavore.

Try this exercise:

The easiest way to get local food is to move away from your local grocers and into the resources that are readily available in your community. This is a beautiful fulfilling habitual shift!

To begin, identify your community resources.

Use Localharvest.org to find Farmer's Markets and learn about CSA options.

Choose a Farmer's Market to visit and purchase your next batch of fresh vegetables.

Where is the closest Farmer's Market?

When will you go?

What do you hope to find?

After your visit, return here to answer the following:

1. **What was your experience like at the market?**

2. **Did you choose to purchase any produce?**

3. **If so, how will you prepare it?**

4. **What did you notice about the produce at the Farmer's Market?**

5. **Will you return? If so, log the next projected visit into your calendar.**

What other action would you like to take in order to move your food choices to be from local resources? Will you tend a garden of your own?

DATE: _____

Morning thoughts:

_____
_____
_____
_____
_____
_____
_____

Food

Water: IIII IIII IIII

Breakfast:
_____
_____

Lunch:
_____
_____
_____

Dinner:
_____
_____
_____

Snacks:
_____
_____
_____

Notes:
_____
_____
_____

Goals & Intentions for today

1
2
3
4
5
6

6:00	
7:00	
8:00	
9:00	
10:00	
11:00	
12:00	
1:00	
2:00	
3:00	
4:00	
5:00	
6:00	
7:00	

Gratitude

REFLECTION

_____
_____
_____
_____
_____
_____

Journal & Schedule

Morning thoughts:
_____
_____
_____
_____
_____
_____
_____

Food

Water: IIII IIII IIII

Breakfast:
_____
_____
_____

Lunch:
_____
_____
_____
_____

Goals & Intentions for today

1
2
3
4
5
6

Dinner:
_____
_____
_____

Snacks:
_____
_____
_____

Notes:
_____
_____
_____

6:00	
7:00	
8:00	
9:00	
10:00	
11:00	
12:00	
1:00	
2:00	
3:00	
4:00	
5:00	
6:00	
7:00	

Gratitude

REFLECTION
_____
_____
_____
_____
_____
_____

DATE: _____

Morning thoughts:
_____
_____
_____
_____
_____
_____
_____

Goals & Intentions for today

1	
2	
3	
4	
5	
6	

6:00	
7:00	
8:00	
9:00	
10:00	
11:00	
12:00	
1:00	
2:00	
3:00	
4:00	
5:00	
6:00	
7:00	

Food

Water: IIII IIII IIII

Breakfast:
_____
_____
_____

Lunch:
_____
_____
_____

Dinner:
_____
_____
_____

Snacks:
_____
_____

Notes:
_____
_____
_____
_____
_____

Gratitude

REFLECTION
_____
_____
_____
_____
_____
_____

Journal & Schedule

Morning thoughts:
_____
_____
_____
_____
_____
_____
_____

Food

Water: IIII IIII IIII

Breakfast:
_____
_____
_____

Lunch:
_____
_____
_____

Dinner:
_____
_____
_____

Snacks:
_____
_____

Notes:
_____
_____
_____

Goals & Intentions for today

1	
2	
3	
4	
5	
6	

6:00	
7:00	
8:00	
9:00	
10:00	
11:00	
12:00	
1:00	
2:00	
3:00	
4:00	
5:00	
6:00	
7:00	

Gratitude

REFLECTION
_____
_____
_____
_____
_____
_____

DATE: _____

Journal & Schedule

Morning thoughts:
_____
_____
_____
_____
_____
_____
_____

Goals & Intentions for today

1
2
3
4
5
6

6:00	
7:00	
8:00	
9:00	
10:00	
11:00	
12:00	
1:00	
2:00	
3:00	
4:00	
5:00	
6:00	
7:00	

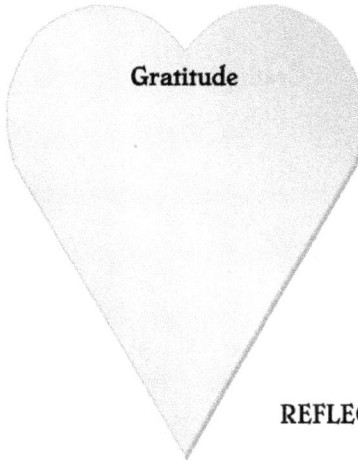

Food

Water: IIII IIII IIII

Breakfast:
_____
_____

Lunch:
_____
_____
_____

Dinner:
_____
_____

Snacks:
_____
_____

Notes:
_____
_____
_____

Gratitude

REFLECTION
_____
_____
_____
_____
_____
_____

DATE: _____

Morning thoughts:
_____
_____
_____
_____
_____
_____
_____

Food

Water: IIII IIII IIII

Breakfast:
_____
_____
_____

Goals & Intentions for today

1

2

3

4

5

6

Lunch:
_____
_____
_____

Dinner:
_____
_____
_____

Snacks:
_____
_____
_____

6:00	
7:00	
8:00	
9:00	
10:00	
11:00	
12:00	
1:00	
2:00	
3:00	
4:00	
5:00	
6:00	
7:00	

Notes:
_____
_____
_____

Gratitude

REFLECTION

_____
_____
_____
_____
_____
_____

Journal & Schedule

Morning thoughts:
_____
_____
_____
_____
_____
_____
_____

Food

Water: IIII IIII IIII

Breakfast:
_____
_____
_____

Lunch:
_____
_____
_____

Dinner:
_____
_____
_____

Snacks:
_____
_____
_____

Notes:
_____
_____
_____

Goals & Intentions for today

1	
2	
3	
4	
5	
6	

6:00	
7:00	
8:00	
9:00	
10:00	
11:00	
12:00	
1:00	
2:00	
3:00	
4:00	
5:00	
6:00	
7:00	

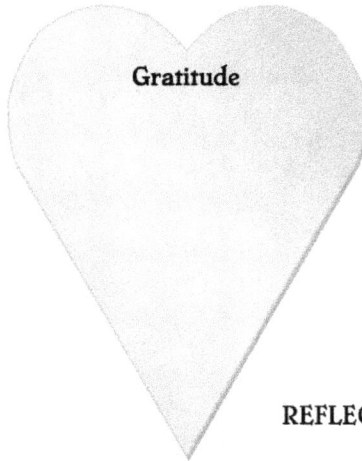

Gratitude

REFLECTION
_____
_____
_____
_____
_____
_____

DATE: _____

Morning thoughts:

_____
_____
_____
_____
_____
_____

Food

Water: IIII IIII IIII

Breakfast:

_____
_____

Goals & Intentions for today

1	
2	
3	
4	
5	
6	

Lunch:

_____
_____

Dinner:

_____
_____

Snacks:

_____
_____

6:00	
7:00	
8:00	
9:00	
10:00	
11:00	
12:00	
1:00	
2:00	
3:00	
4:00	
5:00	
6:00	
7:00	

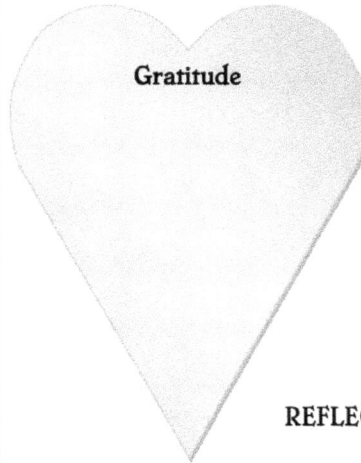

Gratitude

Notes:

_____
_____
_____

REFLECTION

_____
_____
_____
_____
_____

DATE: _____

Morning thoughts:

_____
_____
_____
_____
_____
_____
_____

Goals & Intentions for today

1
2
3
4
5
6

6:00	
7:00	
8:00	
9:00	
10:00	
11:00	
12:00	
1:00	
2:00	
3:00	
4:00	
5:00	
6:00	
7:00	

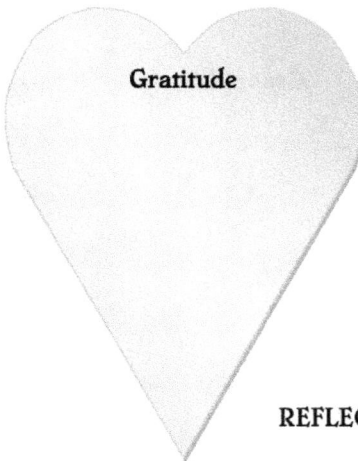

Gratitude

Food

Water: IIII IIII IIII

Breakfast:
_____
_____

Lunch:
_____
_____
_____

Dinner:
_____
_____
_____

Snacks:
_____
_____

Notes:
_____
_____
_____

REFLECTION

_____
_____
_____
_____
_____
_____

DATE: _____

Morning thoughts:
_____
_____
_____
_____
_____
_____
_____

Goals & Intentions for today

1
2
3
4
5
6

6:00	
7:00	
8:00	
9:00	
10:00	
11:00	
12:00	
1:00	
2:00	
3:00	
4:00	
5:00	
6:00	
7:00	

Food

Water: IIII IIII IIII

Breakfast:
_____
_____
_____

Lunch:
_____
_____
_____

Dinner:
_____
_____
_____

Snacks:
_____
_____
_____

Notes:
_____
_____
_____

Gratitude

REFLECTION

_____
_____
_____
_____
_____
_____

237

DATE: _____

Morning thoughts:
_____
_____
_____
_____
_____
_____
_____

Goals & Intentions for today

1	
2	
3	
4	
5	
6	

6:00	
7:00	
8:00	
9:00	
10:00	
11:00	
12:00	
1:00	
2:00	
3:00	
4:00	
5:00	
6:00	
7:00	

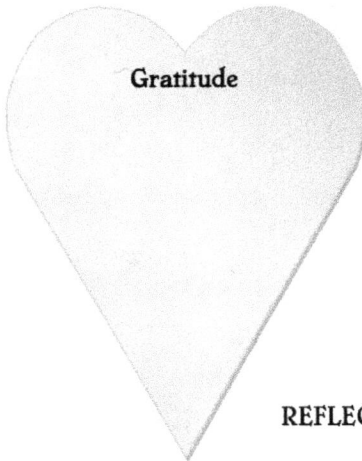

Food

Water: IIII IIII IIII

Breakfast:
_____
_____
_____

Lunch:
_____
_____
_____

Dinner:
_____
_____
_____

Snacks:
_____
_____
_____

Notes:
_____
_____
_____

Gratitude

REFLECTION
_____
_____
_____
_____
_____
_____

238

Journal & Schedule

Morning thoughts:
_____
_____
_____
_____
_____
_____
_____

Goals & Intentions for today

1
2
3
4
5
6

6:00	
7:00	
8:00	
9:00	
10:00	
11:00	
12:00	
1:00	
2:00	
3:00	
4:00	
5:00	
6:00	
7:00	

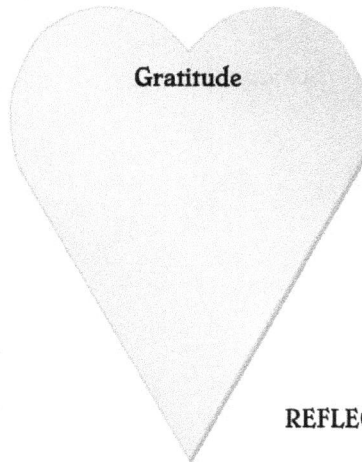

Food

Water: IIII IIII IIII

Breakfast:
_____
_____
_____

Lunch:
_____
_____
_____

Dinner:
_____
_____
_____

Snacks:
_____
_____

Notes:
_____
_____
_____

Gratitude

REFLECTION
_____
_____
_____
_____
_____
_____

DATE: _____

Morning thoughts:
_____
_____
_____
_____
_____
_____
_____

Goals & Intentions for today

1
2
3
4
5
6

6:00	
7:00	
8:00	
9:00	
10:00	
11:00	
12:00	
1:00	
2:00	
3:00	
4:00	
5:00	
6:00	
7:00	

Food

Water: IIII IIII IIII

Breakfast:
_____
_____

Lunch:
_____
_____
_____

Dinner:
_____
_____

Snacks:
_____
_____

Notes:
_____
_____
_____

Gratitude

REFLECTION
_____
_____
_____
_____
_____
_____

DATE: _____

Morning thoughts:
_____
_____
_____
_____
_____
_____
_____

Goals & Intentions for today

1
2
3
4
5
6

6:00	
7:00	
8:00	
9:00	
10:00	
11:00	
12:00	
1:00	
2:00	
3:00	
4:00	
5:00	
6:00	
7:00	

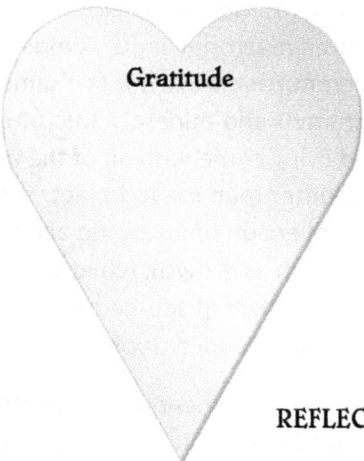

Food

Water: IIII IIII IIII

Breakfast:
_____
_____
_____

Lunch:
_____
_____
_____

Dinner:
_____
_____
_____

Snacks:
_____
_____

Notes:
_____
_____
_____

Gratitude

REFLECTION

_____
_____
_____
_____
_____
_____

Eat Wisely

The most difficult mindset to embrace was a plate that was no longer meat centered. I still eat meat, but when I'm fully listening to and honoring my body, I am only eating it a few times a week and I'm incredibly cautious where it comes from. I feel lighter, my digestion is better, my gut is not bloated, and even my thoughts are more clear.

I can see in my own process and fluctuating needs with this one food group, that everyone is incredibly different, as I myself have different needs almost every day.

--

Protein is a highly controversial topic and one that must be acknowledged on a journey to wellness. There are enormous amounts of conflicting ideas around whether we should or should not consume animal foods.

Some people do really well by including animal foods in their diet; I am one of them. However, I also know that some people do really well by excluding them. Through deep inner exploration and listening closely to your body, you can identify what works best for you. In my practice, we give this topic plenty of space and experimentation. The industry is harsh, unbalanced, and often immoral. As Omnivores, we need to take this into consideration when we choose foods to put into our body.

Protein in itself is a required macronutrient. Macronutrient means basically nutrients we need the most of. Protein, fats, and carbohydrates are the three macronutrients. Almost all living foods contain some combination of all three macronutrients. Macronutrients are not the same as micronutrients. Micronutrients are what you are used to hearing spoken of as vitamins and minerals. Micronutrients basically means what we need in smaller amounts. Foods that are whole and living come with all of the above in some combination. This means that you can get protein from sources of food other than meat. In fact, some plants come very close to mirroring the same sort of complete protein (actually a collection of 13 amino acids), that is found in animal food. The amount you need varies depending on factors such as growth, (children need more per pound of body weight than adults), exercise, (protein is not the body's preferred source of energy, rather it helps the repair and growth of tissue.), age, (older adults need less), and gender. Typically men do better with more than women.

Protein is available in all animal foods including meat, yogurt, butter, milk, and other dairy products. As I've mentioned above, it's also available in plant foods. Quinoa and other grains, beans, legumes, nuts, and seeds are all sources of protein.

While this is a *very* basic illustration of how this nutrient works, I hope it will help you to understand the role protein plays in your wellbeing and that you have choices.

Where does your protein come from? What sources do you choose? What factors do you look for when you choose? Price? Color? Size? Do you read meat labels? Do you seek out sources that are local and more sustainable?

The most healthful options when choosing animal products include:

- ∞ Locally raised/humanely raised
- ∞ Pastured

- ∞ Antibiotic Free
- ∞ Green Finished
- ∞ Grass Fed
- ∞ Wild Caught

Often you can find these options through ranchers and farmers at your local farmers market and CSA. It's important to ask questions and to do your research.

Try this exercise:

As you are learning more about where your food comes from and the implications it has on your health and the environment, the choices you make on a daily basis may begin to naturally shift.

This is a process we call *crowding out*. Have you noticed I have not said you have to eliminate entire food groups? For this journey, you've been setting your own food rules based on your experience and knowledge.

Let this journey continue with what you are learning about your protein sources. Over the next two weeks, experiment with your animal foods. Try noticing how your body feels when you increase and decrease the meat and dairy on your plate. Try experimenting with plant sources of protein such as beans & rice, legumes, soy, and quinoa.

What role does animal food play in your daily meals? (Frequency, serving size, types)

How do you feel after eating animal foods?

What happens if you reduce the amount in a given meal or remove it from one of the three meals each day? How do you feel?

What happens if you increase the amount given in a meal or add it to another meal throughout the day? How do you feel?

What sort of changes would you like to make around this food group?

DATE: _____

Morning thoughts:
_____
_____
_____
_____
_____
_____
_____

Goals & Intentions for today

1
2
3
4
5
6

6:00	
7:00	
8:00	
9:00	
10:00	
11:00	
12:00	
1:00	
2:00	
3:00	
4:00	
5:00	
6:00	
7:00	

Food

Water: IIII IIII IIII

Breakfast:
_____
_____
_____

Lunch:
_____
_____
_____

Dinner:
_____
_____
_____

Snacks:
_____
_____
_____

Notes:
_____
_____
_____

Gratitude

REFLECTION

_____
_____
_____
_____
_____
_____

DATE: _____

Morning thoughts:
_____
_____
_____
_____
_____
_____
_____

Goals & Intentions for today

1
2
3
4
5
6

6:00	
7:00	
8:00	
9:00	
10:00	
11:00	
12:00	
1:00	
2:00	
3:00	
4:00	
5:00	
6:00	
7:00	

Food

Water: IIII IIII IIII

Breakfast:
_____
_____
_____

Lunch:
_____
_____
_____

Dinner:
_____
_____
_____

Snacks:
_____
_____
_____

Notes:
_____
_____
_____

Gratitude

REFLECTION
_____
_____
_____
_____
_____
_____

DATE: _____

Morning thoughts:
_____
_____
_____
_____
_____
_____
_____

Goals & Intentions for today

1	
2	
3	
4	
5	
6	

6:00	
7:00	
8:00	
9:00	
10:00	
11:00	
12:00	
1:00	
2:00	
3:00	
4:00	
5:00	
6:00	
7:00	

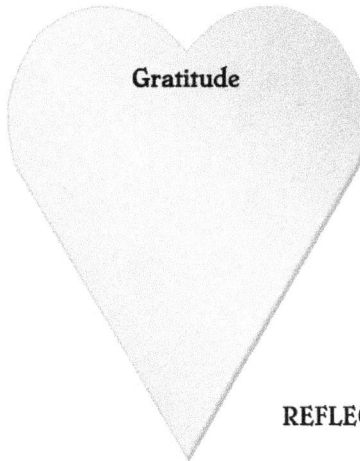

Food

Water: IIII IIII IIII

Breakfast:
_____
_____
_____

Lunch:
_____
_____
_____

Dinner:
_____
_____
_____

Snacks:
_____
_____
_____

Notes:
_____
_____
_____

Gratitude

REFLECTION
_____
_____
_____
_____
_____
_____

Journal & Schedule

Morning thoughts:
_____
_____
_____
_____
_____
_____
_____

Goals & Intentions for today

1
2
3
4
5
6

6:00	
7:00	
8:00	
9:00	
10:00	
11:00	
12:00	
1:00	
2:00	
3:00	
4:00	
5:00	
6:00	
7:00	

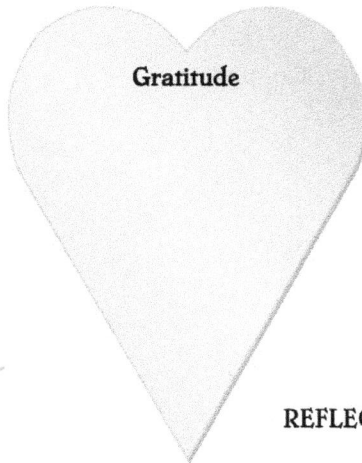

Food

Water: IIII IIII IIII

Breakfast:
_____
_____
_____

Lunch:
_____
_____
_____

Dinner:
_____
_____
_____

Snacks:
_____
_____

Notes:
_____
_____
_____
_____

Gratitude

REFLECTION
_____
_____
_____
_____
_____

DATE: _____

Morning thoughts:

_____
_____
_____
_____
_____
_____
_____

Food

Water: IIII IIII IIII

Breakfast:
_____
_____
_____

Goals & Intentions for today

1	
2	
3	
4	
5	
6	

Lunch:
_____
_____
_____

Dinner:
_____
_____
_____

Snacks:
_____
_____
_____

6:00	
7:00	
8:00	
9:00	
10:00	
11:00	
12:00	
1:00	
2:00	
3:00	
4:00	
5:00	
6:00	
7:00	

Notes:
_____
_____
_____

Gratitude

REFLECTION

_____
_____
_____
_____
_____
_____

DATE: _____

Morning thoughts:

_____
_____
_____
_____
_____
_____
_____

Goals & Intentions for today

1
2
3
4
5
6

6:00	
7:00	
8:00	
9:00	
10:00	
11:00	
12:00	
1:00	
2:00	
3:00	
4:00	
5:00	
6:00	
7:00	

Gratitude

Food

Water: IIII IIII IIII

Breakfast:
_____
_____
_____

Lunch:
_____
_____
_____

Dinner:
_____
_____
_____

Snacks:
_____
_____
_____

Notes:
_____
_____

REFLECTION

_____
_____
_____
_____
_____
_____

249

DATE: _____

Morning thoughts:
_____
_____
_____
_____
_____
_____
_____

Food

Water: IIII IIII IIII

Breakfast:
_____
_____
_____

Lunch:
_____
_____
_____

Dinner:
_____
_____
_____

Snacks:
_____
_____
_____

Notes:
_____
_____
_____

Goals & Intentions for today

1

2

3

4

5

6

6:00	
7:00	
8:00	
9:00	
10:00	
11:00	
12:00	
1:00	
2:00	
3:00	
4:00	
5:00	
6:00	
7:00	

Gratitude

REFLECTION
_____
_____
_____
_____
_____
_____

DATE: _____

Morning thoughts:

_____
_____
_____
_____
_____
_____
_____

Food

Water: IIII IIII IIII

Breakfast:
_____
_____
_____

Goals & Intentions for today

1	
2	
3	
4	
5	
6	

Lunch:
_____
_____
_____

Dinner:
_____
_____
_____

Snacks:
_____
_____

6:00	
7:00	
8:00	
9:00	
10:00	
11:00	
12:00	
1:00	
2:00	
3:00	
4:00	
5:00	
6:00	
7:00	

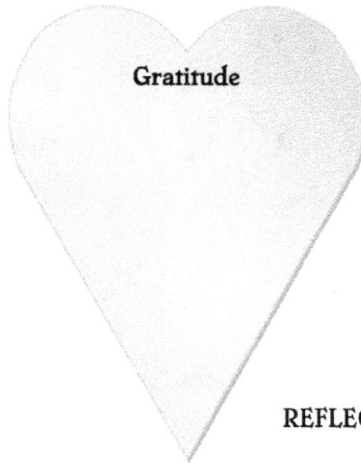

Notes:
_____
_____
_____

Gratitude

REFLECTION

_____
_____
_____
_____
_____
_____

DATE: _____

Morning thoughts:
_____
_____
_____
_____
_____
_____
_____

Food

Water: IIII IIII IIII

Breakfast:
_____
_____
_____

Goals & Intentions for today

1
2
3
4
5
6

Lunch:
_____
_____
_____

Dinner:
_____
_____
_____

Snacks:
_____
_____
_____

6:00	
7:00	
8:00	
9:00	
10:00	
11:00	
12:00	
1:00	
2:00	
3:00	
4:00	
5:00	
6:00	
7:00	

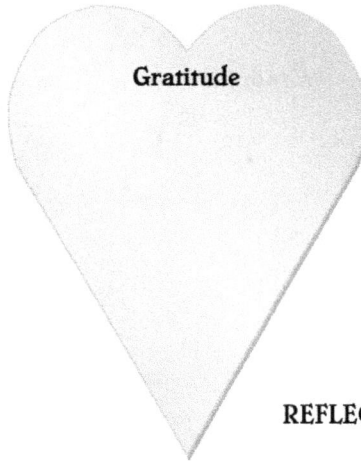

Gratitude

Notes:
_____
_____
_____

REFLECTION

_____
_____
_____
_____
_____
_____

DATE: _____

Morning thoughts:
_____
_____
_____
_____
_____
_____
_____

Goals & Intentions for today

1
2
3
4
5
6

6:00	
7:00	
8:00	
9:00	
10:00	
11:00	
12:00	
1:00	
2:00	
3:00	
4:00	
5:00	
6:00	
7:00	

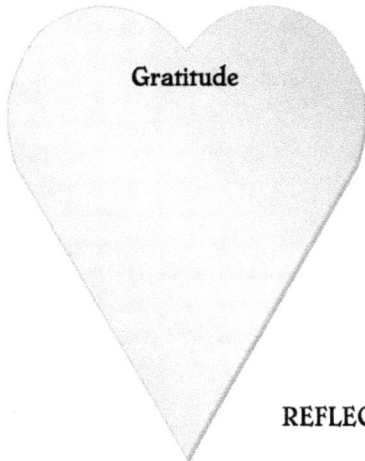

Food

Water: IIII IIII IIII

Breakfast:
_____
_____
_____

Lunch:
_____
_____
_____

Dinner:
_____
_____
_____

Snacks:
_____
_____
_____

Notes:
_____
_____
_____

Gratitude

REFLECTION

_____
_____
_____
_____
_____
_____

253

DATE: _____

Morning thoughts:
_____
_____
_____
_____
_____
_____
_____

Food

Water: IIII IIII IIII

Breakfast:
_____
_____
_____

Goals & Intentions for today

1	
2	
3	
4	
5	
6	

Lunch:
_____
_____
_____

Dinner:
_____
_____
_____

Snacks:
_____
_____

6:00	
7:00	
8:00	
9:00	
10:00	
11:00	
12:00	
1:00	
2:00	
3:00	
4:00	
5:00	
6:00	
7:00	

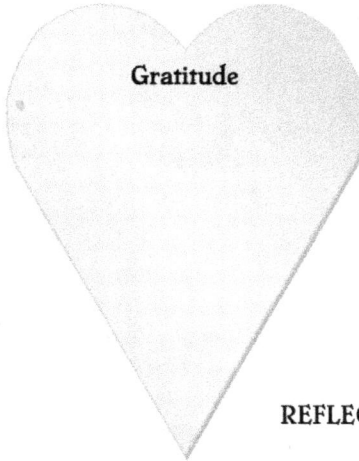

Notes:
_____
_____
_____
_____

Gratitude

REFLECTION
_____
_____
_____
_____
_____
_____

DATE: _____

Morning thoughts:
_____
_____
_____
_____
_____
_____
_____

Food

Water: IIII IIII IIII

Breakfast:
_____
_____
_____

Goals & Intentions for today

1
2
3
4
5
6

Lunch:
_____
_____
_____

Dinner:
_____
_____
_____

Snacks:
_____
_____

6:00	
7:00	
8:00	
9:00	
10:00	
11:00	
12:00	
1:00	
2:00	
3:00	
4:00	
5:00	
6:00	
7:00	

Notes:
_____
_____

Gratitude

REFLECTION

_____
_____
_____
_____
_____
_____

DATE: _____

Morning thoughts:
_____
_____
_____
_____
_____
_____
_____

Food

Water: IIII IIII IIII

Breakfast:
_____
_____

Goals & Intentions for today

1	
2	
3	
4	
5	
6	

Lunch:
_____
_____
_____

Dinner:
_____
_____
_____

Snacks:
_____
_____

6:00	
7:00	
8:00	
9:00	
10:00	
11:00	
12:00	
1:00	
2:00	
3:00	
4:00	
5:00	
6:00	
7:00	

Notes:
_____
_____
_____
_____

Gratitude

REFLECTION
_____
_____
_____
_____
_____
_____

DATE: _____

Morning thoughts:
_____
_____
_____
_____
_____
_____
_____

Goals & Intentions for today

1
2
3
4
5
6

6:00	
7:00	
8:00	
9:00	
10:00	
11:00	
12:00	
1:00	
2:00	
3:00	
4:00	
5:00	
6:00	
7:00	

Food

Water: IIII IIII IIII

Breakfast:
_____
_____
_____

Lunch:
_____
_____
_____

Dinner:
_____
_____
_____

Snacks:
_____
_____
_____

Notes:
_____
_____
_____

Gratitude

REFLECTION
_____
_____
_____
_____
_____

Eat Prebiotics & Probiotics

"If you sit on a tack, you don't take an aspirin to take away the pain, you take out the tack!" – Susan Blum, MD, MPH

I'm sitting in my GI Specialist's office listening to the words that are coming out of his mouth, feeling self-conscious and sitting with the idea that this guy has seen parts of me I haven't and that we are talking about things I don't want to be talking about – my bowels.

His general demeanor is as if it's just another day's Irritable Bowel Syndrome diagnosis. He says something to the effect of, "There isn't much you can do, there's not really a cure for this that we know of. There does seem to be some link with stress, so you can focus on eliminating stress in your life." I roll my eyes. My job is the first thing that comes to my mind. Then he continues, "I have a medication you can try, if you'd like."

My head is spinning. What does he mean there isn't much I can do? There's medication? What does he mean by eliminate stress? What am I supposed to do, quit my job? Ha! Ha! Jokes on me!

--

In time, I did heal my IBS. I found that stress played a significant role, but the food did too. There are a lot of dietary theories circulating today that address IBS. Many are amazing and helpful. Most have a common factor. Eat natural, whole foods, and include probiotics in the mix. It turns out that including probiotics in our diet may in fact support a healthy digestive tract. As an industry, this idea has caught on and spread like a wild fire in dead timber. There are pills and potions, every possible flavor of sugary sweetened yogurt, and even guidelines on what pills make it how far in your digestive tract.

I began including prebiotics and probiotics in my diet as a part of the healing nutritional changes I was making when I was a student, yet I remained focused and committed to the idea of the whole foods approach.

--

My favorite probiotics are:

1. Fermented vegetables: sounds awful but think sauerkraut and kimchi – the canned, on the shelf, variety do not work for this application, rather seek out refrigerated raw, or make your own.
2. Yogurt: Not just any – try organic, grass fed, plain
3. Good Belly Straight Shot (low sugar, dairy free)

Prebiotics are:

These are foods that cannot be digested by the digestive tract. They ferment and become food for the probiotic. Probiotic means "for life" and these are natural bacteria that live in your digestive tract that help to control bad bacteria. Including a probiotic will help to replenish the good bacteria in your gut. Prebiotics are present in whole grains like rice, quinoa, and oats as well as vegetables like leeks, artichokes, onions, and bananas.

<u>Try this exercise:</u>

Consider the amount of new foods you are now including in your daily diet that may serve as prebiotic foods. How about probiotic foods?

Which of these would you like to add on a regular basis?

Choose one or two ways to improve your prebiotic and probiotic intake.

Try to include these daily for two weeks, tracking your experience on the journal pages in this workbook.

After two weeks, return to report your results.

What did you notice about including these foods in your diet?

How is your digestion? Bowel Movements? Sleep? Focus? Energy?

What is your favorite probiotic? Why?

Journal & Schedule

Morning thoughts:
_____
_____
_____
_____
_____
_____
_____

Goals & Intentions for today

1
2
3
4
5
6

6:00	
7:00	
8:00	
9:00	
10:00	
11:00	
12:00	
1:00	
2:00	
3:00	
4:00	
5:00	
6:00	
7:00	

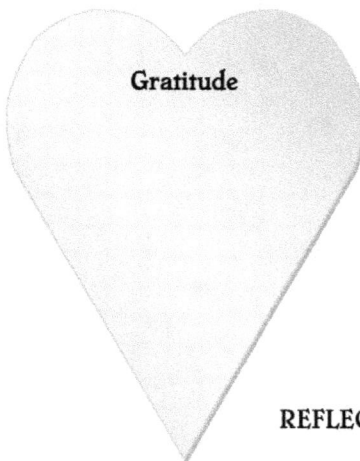

Gratitude

Food

Water: IIII IIII IIII

Breakfast:
_____
_____
_____

Lunch:
_____
_____
_____

Dinner:
_____
_____
_____

Snacks:
_____
_____
_____

Notes:
_____
_____
_____

REFLECTION
_____
_____
_____
_____
_____
_____

DATE: _____

Morning thoughts:
_____
_____
_____
_____
_____
_____
_____

Food

Water: IIII IIII IIII

Breakfast:
_____
_____
_____

Goals & Intentions for today

1
2
3
4
5
6

Lunch:
_____
_____
_____
_____

Dinner:
_____
_____
_____

Snacks:
_____
_____

Notes:
_____
_____
_____
_____

6:00	
7:00	
8:00	
9:00	
10:00	
11:00	
12:00	
1:00	
2:00	
3:00	
4:00	
5:00	
6:00	
7:00	

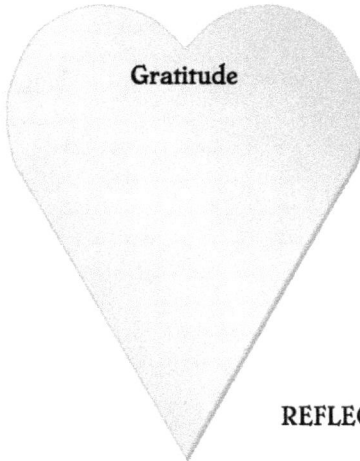

Gratitude

REFLECTION
_____
_____
_____
_____
_____
_____

DATE: _____

Morning thoughts:
_____
_____
_____
_____
_____
_____
_____

Food

Water: IIII IIII IIII

Breakfast:
_____
_____
_____

Lunch:
_____
_____
_____

Goals & Intentions for today

1	
2	
3	
4	
5	
6	

Dinner:
_____
_____
_____

Snacks:
_____
_____

Notes:
_____
_____
_____
_____

6:00	
7:00	
8:00	
9:00	
10:00	
11:00	
12:00	
1:00	
2:00	
3:00	
4:00	
5:00	
6:00	
7:00	

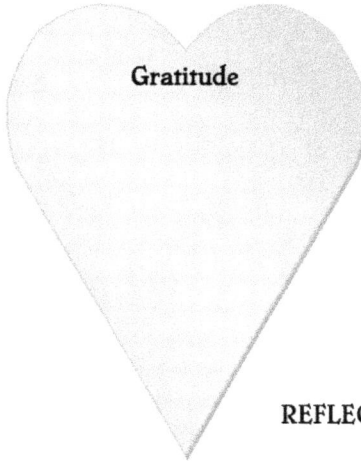

Gratitude

REFLECTION
_____
_____
_____
_____
_____
_____

Journal & Schedule

Morning thoughts:
_____
_____
_____
_____
_____
_____
_____

Goals & Intentions for today

1
2
3
4
5
6

6:00	
7:00	
8:00	
9:00	
10:00	
11:00	
12:00	
1:00	
2:00	
3:00	
4:00	
5:00	
6:00	
7:00	

Food

Water: IIII IIII IIII

Breakfast:
_____
_____
_____

Lunch:
_____
_____
_____

Dinner:
_____
_____
_____

Snacks:
_____
_____
_____

Notes:
_____
_____
_____

Gratitude

REFLECTION
_____
_____
_____
_____
_____
_____

DATE: _____

Morning thoughts:
_____
_____
_____
_____
_____
_____
_____

Food

Water: IIII IIII IIII

Breakfast:
_____
_____
_____

Goals & Intentions for today

1	
2	
3	
4	
5	
6	

Lunch:
_____
_____
_____

Dinner:
_____
_____
_____

Snacks:
_____
_____
_____

6:00	
7:00	
8:00	
9:00	
10:00	
11:00	
12:00	
1:00	
2:00	
3:00	
4:00	
5:00	
6:00	
7:00	

Notes:
_____
_____
_____

Gratitude

REFLECTION

_____
_____
_____
_____
_____
_____

DATE: _____

Morning thoughts:
_____
_____
_____
_____
_____
_____
_____

Goals & Intentions for today

1
2
3
4
5
6

6:00	
7:00	
8:00	
9:00	
10:00	
11:00	
12:00	
1:00	
2:00	
3:00	
4:00	
5:00	
6:00	
7:00	

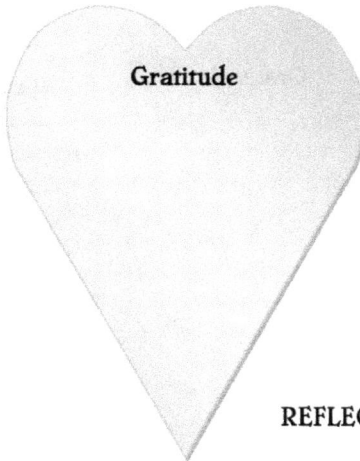

Food

Water: IIII IIII IIII

Breakfast:
_____
_____
_____

Lunch:
_____
_____
_____

Dinner:
_____
_____
_____

Snacks:
_____
_____
_____

Notes:
_____
_____

Gratitude

REFLECTION

_____
_____
_____
_____
_____
_____

Journal & Schedule

Morning thoughts:
_____
_____
_____
_____
_____
_____
_____

Food

Water: IIII IIII IIII

Breakfast:
_____
_____
_____

Goals & Intentions for today

1	
2	
3	
4	
5	
6	

Lunch:
_____
_____
_____

Dinner:
_____
_____
_____

6:00	
7:00	
8:00	
9:00	
10:00	
11:00	
12:00	
1:00	
2:00	
3:00	
4:00	
5:00	
6:00	
7:00	

Snacks:
_____
_____
_____

Notes:
_____
_____
_____

Gratitude

REFLECTION

_____
_____
_____
_____
_____
_____

DATE: _____

Morning thoughts:

_____
_____
_____
_____
_____
_____
_____

Food

Water: IIII IIII IIII

Breakfast:

_____
_____
_____

Goals & Intentions for today

1
2
3
4
5
6

Lunch:

_____
_____
_____

Dinner:

_____
_____
_____

Snacks:

_____
_____
_____

6:00	
7:00	
8:00	
9:00	
10:00	
11:00	
12:00	
1:00	
2:00	
3:00	
4:00	
5:00	
6:00	
7:00	

Notes:

_____
_____
_____

Gratitude

REFLECTION

_____
_____
_____
_____
_____
_____

DATE: _____

Morning thoughts:
_____
_____
_____
_____
_____
_____
_____

Goals & Intentions for today

1
2
3
4
5
6

6:00	
7:00	
8:00	
9:00	
10:00	
11:00	
12:00	
1:00	
2:00	
3:00	
4:00	
5:00	
6:00	
7:00	

Food

Water: IIII IIII IIII

Breakfast:
_____
_____

Lunch:
_____
_____
_____

Dinner:
_____
_____
_____

Snacks:
_____
_____

Notes:
_____
_____
_____
_____

Gratitude

REFLECTION

_____
_____
_____
_____
_____
_____

DATE: _____

Morning thoughts:
_____
_____
_____
_____
_____
_____
_____

Goals & Intentions for today

1
2
3
4
5
6

6:00	
7:00	
8:00	
9:00	
10:00	
11:00	
12:00	
1:00	
2:00	
3:00	
4:00	
5:00	
6:00	
7:00	

Food

Water: IIII IIII IIII

Breakfast:
_____
_____
_____

Lunch:
_____
_____
_____

Dinner:
_____
_____
_____

Snacks:
_____
_____
_____

Notes:
_____
_____
_____
_____

Gratitude

REFLECTION
_____
_____
_____
_____
_____
_____

DATE: _____

Morning thoughts:
_____
_____
_____
_____
_____
_____

Goals & Intentions for today

| 1 |
| 2 |
| 3 |
| 4 |
| 5 |
| 6 |

6:00	
7:00	
8:00	
9:00	
10:00	
11:00	
12:00	
1:00	
2:00	
3:00	
4:00	
5:00	
6:00	
7:00	

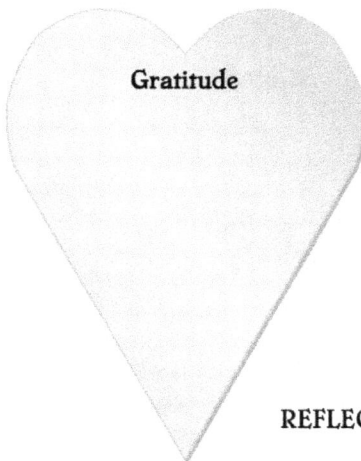

Gratitude

REFLECTION

_____
_____
_____
_____
_____
_____

Food

Water: IIII IIII IIII

Breakfast:
_____
_____
_____

Lunch:
_____
_____
_____

Dinner:
_____
_____
_____

Snacks:
_____
_____
_____

Notes:
_____
_____
_____

DATE: _____

Morning thoughts:
_____
_____
_____
_____
_____
_____
_____

Food

Water: IIII IIII IIII

Breakfast:
_____
_____
_____

Goals & Intentions for today

1	
2	
3	
4	
5	
6	

Lunch:
_____
_____
_____

Dinner:
_____
_____
_____

Snacks:
_____
_____

Notes:
_____
_____
_____

6:00	
7:00	
8:00	
9:00	
10:00	
11:00	
12:00	
1:00	
2:00	
3:00	
4:00	
5:00	
6:00	
7:00	

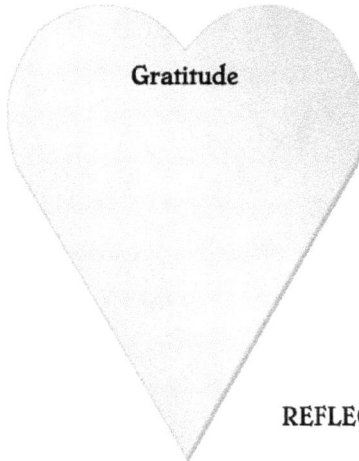

Gratitude

REFLECTION
_____
_____
_____
_____
_____
_____
_____

DATE: _____

Morning thoughts:
_____
_____
_____
_____
_____
_____
_____

Goals & Intentions for today

1	
2	
3	
4	
5	
6	

6:00	
7:00	
8:00	
9:00	
10:00	
11:00	
12:00	
1:00	
2:00	
3:00	
4:00	
5:00	
6:00	
7:00	

Food

Water: IIII IIII IIII

Breakfast:
_____
_____
_____

Lunch:
_____
_____
_____
_____

Dinner:
_____
_____
_____

Snacks:
_____
_____
_____

Notes:
_____
_____
_____

Gratitude

REFLECTION
_____
_____
_____
_____
_____
_____

DATE: _____

Morning thoughts:
_____
_____
_____
_____
_____
_____
_____

Food

Water: IIII IIII IIII

Breakfast:
_____
_____
_____

Goals & Intentions for today

1
2
3
4
5
6

Lunch:
_____
_____
_____

Dinner:
_____
_____
_____

Snacks:
_____
_____

Notes:
_____
_____
_____

6:00	
7:00	
8:00	
9:00	
10:00	
11:00	
12:00	
1:00	
2:00	
3:00	
4:00	
5:00	
6:00	
7:00	

Gratitude

REFLECTION
_____
_____
_____
_____
_____
_____

Eat Colorfully

We are in the line at the checkout and I'm watching the progression of groceries make their way from my cart to the scanner, then to the belt to be bagged. I'm feeling a little dazed, tired, and am only half way paying attention. I hear "bleep…..bleep", I'm watching as the food rolls by…. cheese dip …… bagels … "bleep"… spinach…sandwich bread…."bleep" .. cookies…..hair spray… boxed rice…. "bleep"…. Oreos…. " bleep".. a family sized bag of chips…."bleep"… and I think only that I got a lot. I did not notice how most of the foods I see rolling by weren't on my list, and that they were nearly all packaged and processed.

**Making healthy choices at the grocers takes
practice, presence, and planning.**

Grocery stores are designed to encourage you to shop, if you follow mindlessly, you'll find yourself in the chip and soda isles without even thinking about it!

Before you walk through those grocery store doors, take a moment to drop everything you have in your mind. **Take a deep breath and get present.** Remember that you are walking into a mass media message filled environment where people have spent billions of dollars to hook you into buying products that are not good for you. Start in the produce section and work your way around the outer perimeter of the store. Use a list. **Practice choosing whole foods that fill the many colors of the rainbow.** When you are done and before you check out, review the items you chose to verify that you've chosen what serves you! Are they mostly whole, natural foods? Are they a variety of colors? If so, pat yourself on the back and go home! If not, take a moment to set those extras aside. I used to feel guilty for doing this, but now, I know it's just me stepping back into my body and taking charge. **Will you take charge?**

In my practice, I work with my clients to learn how to read labels. We talk about choosing foods that have five or fewer ingredients and to watch for those with ingredients that we actually understand. I encourage them to reduce sugar grams and to watch for sneaky marketing messages. It's a process, but one you can easily skirt by simply buying foods that don't need a label at all. **Whole foods do not need labels.**

Eat whole most of the time and you've got this part in the bag!

Try this exercise:

For the next two weeks, identify your food plan.

What do you have already in your fridge and cabinets? What are a few ideas you have for what you can make using these ingredients? What will you need to get from the store in order to make these full recipes? If needed, do some research. I love Pinterest as a fun and visually stimulating way to find recipes. (Careful, this can be a time suck!) I also subscribe to food focused magazines like Mother Earth Living, Clean Eating, and Vegetarian Times.

Once you have your plan set, identify the ingredients you do not have in order to make the recipes you'd like to make.

Make your shopping list from this.

Then go shopping!

Before you enter the store, stop to breathe. Get present in your body. Remember to stick to your list. As you choose foods from the produce section, notice options you have. As you choose, identify ways you can upgrade your selections. Is organic better? Is there a fresher version? Is there a different colored, (insert vegetable), that you've never tried?

Before checking out, stop to check your cart.

Did you get anything that wasn't on the list? If so, what? Why? How will you choose to act?

After your shopping trip, answer these questions:

- What went well?

- How did it feel to shop this way?

- What did you notice during your shopping trip?

- What felt challenging?

- What did you learn?

- What will you do differently next time?

P.S. This is a practice that takes time to embrace. It can feel time consuming in the beginning. Often my clients plan too many meals, so it can actually be a little more expensive as you learn how much to plan for.

Stick with it, be patient, slow down, and think it through. In the end, you'll find your way through this, it won't take as much time and you'll end up saving a lot of money.

Through the process of label reading, you'll find brands and products you trust and can return to time after time. All of this will flow with consistent practice, and your body will thank you!

Journal & Schedule

Morning thoughts:

_____
_____
_____
_____
_____
_____
_____

Goals & Intentions for today

1
2
3
4
5
6

6:00	
7:00	
8:00	
9:00	
10:00	
11:00	
12:00	
1:00	
2:00	
3:00	
4:00	
5:00	
6:00	
7:00	

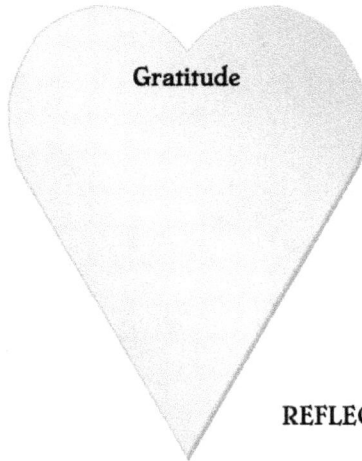

Food

Water: IIII IIII IIII

Breakfast:
_____
_____
_____

Lunch:
_____
_____
_____

Dinner:
_____
_____
_____

Snacks:
_____
_____
_____

Notes:
_____
_____
_____

Gratitude

REFLECTION

_____
_____
_____
_____
_____
_____

DATE: _____

Morning thoughts:

_____
_____
_____
_____
_____
_____
_____

Goals & Intentions for today

1	
2	
3	
4	
5	
6	

6:00	
7:00	
8:00	
9:00	
10:00	
11:00	
12:00	
1:00	
2:00	
3:00	
4:00	
5:00	
6:00	
7:00	

Food

Water: IIII IIII IIII

Breakfast:
_____
_____
_____

Lunch:
_____
_____
_____

Dinner:
_____
_____
_____

Snacks:
_____
_____
_____

Notes:
_____
_____
_____

Gratitude

REFLECTION

_____
_____
_____
_____
_____
_____

DATE: _____

Journal & Schedule

Morning thoughts:
_____
_____
_____
_____
_____
_____
_____

Goals & Intentions for today

1
2
3
4
5
6

6:00	
7:00	
8:00	
9:00	
10:00	
11:00	
12:00	
1:00	
2:00	
3:00	
4:00	
5:00	
6:00	
7:00	

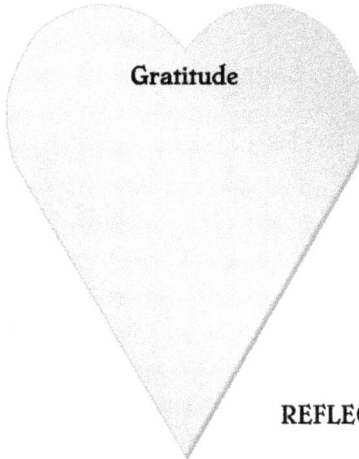

Food

Water: IIII IIII IIII

Breakfast:
_____
_____
_____

Lunch:
_____
_____
_____

Dinner:
_____
_____
_____

Snacks:
_____
_____
_____

Notes:
_____
_____
_____

Gratitude

REFLECTION
_____
_____
_____
_____
_____

DATE: _____

Morning thoughts:
_____
_____
_____
_____
_____
_____
_____

Food

Water: IIII IIII IIII

Breakfast:
_____
_____
_____

Goals & Intentions for today

| 1 |
| 2 |
| 3 |
| 4 |
| 5 |
| 6 |

Lunch:
_____
_____
_____

Dinner:
_____
_____
_____

Snacks:
_____
_____

Notes:
_____
_____
_____

6:00	
7:00	
8:00	
9:00	
10:00	
11:00	
12:00	
1:00	
2:00	
3:00	
4:00	
5:00	
6:00	
7:00	

Gratitude

REFLECTION
_____
_____
_____
_____
_____

DATE: _____

Morning thoughts:
_____
_____
_____
_____
_____
_____
_____
_____

Goals & Intentions for today

1
2
3
4
5
6

6:00	
7:00	
8:00	
9:00	
10:00	
11:00	
12:00	
1:00	
2:00	
3:00	
4:00	
5:00	
6:00	
7:00	

Food

Water: IIII IIII IIII

Breakfast:
_____
_____
_____

Lunch:
_____
_____
_____

Dinner:
_____
_____
_____

Snacks:
_____
_____
_____

Notes:
_____
_____
_____

Gratitude

REFLECTION
_____
_____
_____
_____
_____
_____

DATE: _____

Morning thoughts:

_____
_____
_____
_____
_____
_____
_____
_____

Goals & Intentions for today

1
2
3
4
5
6

6:00	
7:00	
8:00	
9:00	
10:00	
11:00	
12:00	
1:00	
2:00	
3:00	
4:00	
5:00	
6:00	
7:00	

Food

Water: IIII IIII IIII

Breakfast:
_____
_____
_____

Lunch:
_____
_____
_____

Dinner:
_____
_____
_____

Snacks:
_____
_____

Notes:
_____
_____
_____

Gratitude

REFLECTION

_____
_____
_____
_____
_____
_____

DATE: _____

Morning thoughts:
_____
_____
_____
_____
_____
_____
_____

Food

Water: IIII IIII IIII

Breakfast:
_____
_____
_____

Goals & Intentions for today

1	
2	
3	
4	
5	
6	

Lunch:
_____
_____
_____

Dinner:
_____
_____
_____

Snacks:
_____
_____

6:00	
7:00	
8:00	
9:00	
10:00	
11:00	
12:00	
1:00	
2:00	
3:00	
4:00	
5:00	
6:00	
7:00	

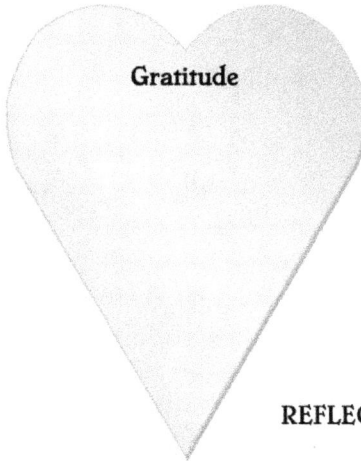

Notes:
_____
_____
_____

Gratitude

REFLECTION
_____
_____
_____
_____
_____
_____

Journal & Schedule

Morning thoughts:

_____
_____
_____
_____
_____
_____
_____

Goals & Intentions for today

1
2
3
4
5
6

6:00	
7:00	
8:00	
9:00	
10:00	
11:00	
12:00	
1:00	
2:00	
3:00	
4:00	
5:00	
6:00	
7:00	

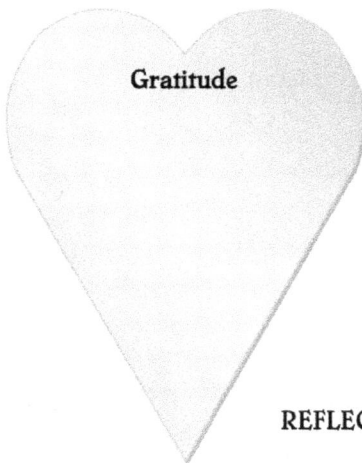

Food

Water: IIII IIII IIII

Breakfast:
_____
_____
_____

Lunch:
_____
_____
_____

Dinner:
_____
_____
_____

Snacks:
_____
_____
_____

Notes:
_____
_____
_____
_____

Gratitude

REFLECTION

_____
_____
_____
_____
_____
_____

DATE: _____

Food

Morning thoughts:
_____
_____
_____
_____
_____
_____
_____

Water: IIII IIII IIII

Breakfast:
_____
_____
_____

Goals & Intentions for today

1	
2	
3	
4	
5	
6	

Lunch:
_____
_____
_____

Dinner:
_____
_____
_____

Snacks:
_____
_____
_____

6:00	
7:00	
8:00	
9:00	
10:00	
11:00	
12:00	
1:00	
2:00	
3:00	
4:00	
5:00	
6:00	
7:00	

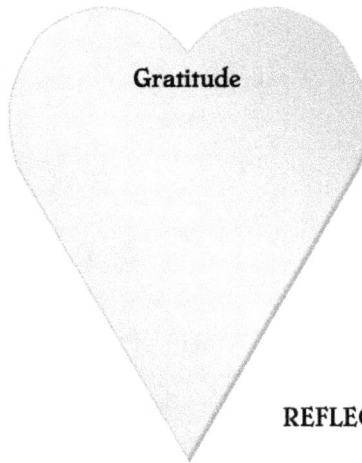

Notes:
_____
_____
_____
_____

Gratitude

REFLECTION

_____
_____
_____
_____
_____
_____

Journal & Schedule

Morning thoughts:

_____
_____
_____
_____
_____
_____
_____

Goals & Intentions for today

1
2
3
4
5
6

6:00	
7:00	
8:00	
9:00	
10:00	
11:00	
12:00	
1:00	
2:00	
3:00	
4:00	
5:00	
6:00	
7:00	

Food

Water: IIII IIII IIII

Breakfast:
_____
_____
_____

Lunch:
_____
_____
_____

Dinner:
_____
_____
_____

Snacks:
_____
_____
_____

Notes:
_____
_____
_____

Gratitude

REFLECTION

_____
_____
_____
_____
_____
_____

DATE: _____

Morning thoughts:
_____
_____
_____
_____
_____
_____

Goals & Intentions for today

1
2
3
4
5
6

6:00	
7:00	
8:00	
9:00	
10:00	
11:00	
12:00	
1:00	
2:00	
3:00	
4:00	
5:00	
6:00	
7:00	

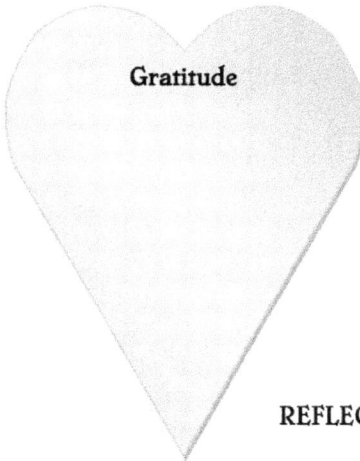

Food

Water: IIII IIII IIII

Breakfast:
_____
_____
_____

Lunch:
_____
_____
_____

Dinner:
_____
_____
_____

Snacks:
_____
_____
_____

Notes:
_____
_____
_____

Gratitude

REFLECTION
_____
_____
_____
_____
_____
_____

DATE: _____

Morning thoughts:
_____
_____
_____
_____
_____
_____
_____

Goals & Intentions for today

1	
2	
3	
4	
5	
6	

6:00	
7:00	
8:00	
9:00	
10:00	
11:00	
12:00	
1:00	
2:00	
3:00	
4:00	
5:00	
6:00	
7:00	

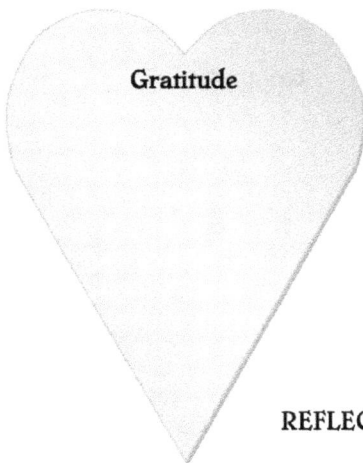

Food

Water: IIII IIII IIII

Breakfast:
_____
_____
_____

Lunch:
_____
_____
_____

Dinner:
_____
_____
_____

Snacks:
_____
_____
_____

Notes:
_____
_____
_____

Gratitude

REFLECTION
_____
_____
_____
_____
_____
_____

DATE: _____

Morning thoughts:
_____
_____
_____
_____
_____
_____
_____

Food

Water: IIII IIII IIII

Breakfast:
_____
_____
_____

Goals & Intentions for today

1

2

3

4

5

6

Lunch:
_____
_____
_____

Dinner:
_____
_____
_____

Snacks:
_____
_____
_____

6:00	
7:00	
8:00	
9:00	
10:00	
11:00	
12:00	
1:00	
2:00	
3:00	
4:00	
5:00	
6:00	
7:00	

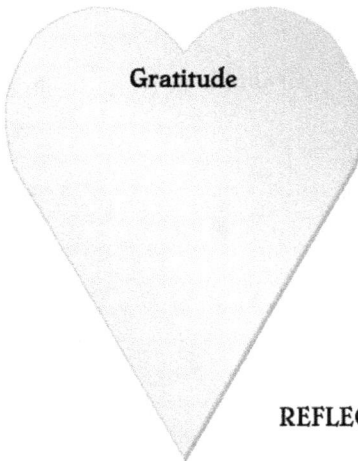

Notes:
_____
_____
_____

Gratitude

REFLECTION

_____
_____
_____
_____
_____
_____

DATE: _____

Morning thoughts:
_____
_____
_____
_____
_____
_____
_____

Goals & Intentions for today

1
2
3
4
5
6

6:00	
7:00	
8:00	
9:00	
10:00	
11:00	
12:00	
1:00	
2:00	
3:00	
4:00	
5:00	
6:00	
7:00	

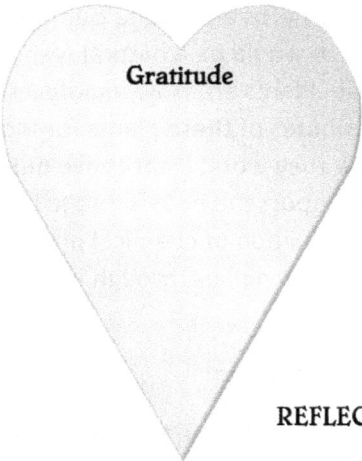

Gratitude

Food

Water: IIII IIII IIII

Breakfast:
_____
_____
_____

Lunch:
_____
_____
_____

Dinner:
_____
_____
_____

Snacks:
_____
_____

Notes:
_____
_____
_____

Journal & Schedule

REFLECTION
_____
_____
_____
_____
_____
_____

Part III – MomPositive Apothecary

Years before I ever thought to attend The Institute for Integrative Nutrition™, I felt really uninspired and unfulfilled. I had been looking outward for satisfaction and happiness, so much so that I was pushing on my husband for entertainment and fulfillment that he simply could not deliver. He suggested I find an interest. What did I want to learn about? What was interesting to me? Maybe a hobby? He made a few suggestions that were relative to what he noticed, I liked to garden, perhaps there was something there that I could pursue. My husband is so smart.

Our location hindered me from taking classes in person, so I found a distance course. Herbalism 101. Something to experiment with, I thought. And so began my journey into the realm of natural healing. By 2005 I completed a diploma program for Master Herbalism from The Australasian College, now the American College of Health Sciences. This was just the gateway to my now continuing education in natural healing.

Today, I hold diplomas and certificates in Holistic Nutrition, Integrative Nutrition Health Coaching, Sports Nutrition, Herbalism and Aromatherapy. My education continues, and I hope always will.

--

Introducing herbs and essential oils into your home can be a fun and sensual way to add depth to your personal care plan. Oils and herbs are beautiful, aromatic, and interesting to learn about.

The biggest mistake we can make is to compare herbs and oils to our modern pharmaceutical medicines. Of course, for most, it's our only experience and so would be a natural response. Yet nature's remedies are dynamically different than those made in a lab. Plants are truly multifaceted gifts of nature. As much as we have tried to break down the components and attributes of these plants for food and healing, we are just beginning to understand how complex they are and how they work. Plants have nutrients and components that work synergistically, intelligently, and naturally to support the body's innate healing abilities. Herbs are simply plants with noted healing properties. Before the introduction of chemical pharmaceuticals in the past 150 years, our forefathers (and mothers) relied on these plants to pull us through events such as plague, chronic disease, and injuries of all kinds.

The history of plants as medicines is vast and fascinating!

My intention for this portion of this workbook is to encourage you to experiment with herbs and essential oils and to take notice of how your body responds to them. It is not by any means a complete guide, simply a gentle introduction with a few ideas. By no means is this a replacement for conventional treatment. (Believe me, modern medicine is a miracle, and has its place too!) If you are taking any medications or are currently suffering from a serious medical condition, please see your doctor before adding herbs or essential oils to your self-care regimen.

If they work well for you, having them on hand can be a quick and empowering way to take charge of you and your family's health and wellbeing. When partnered with the MomPositive Lifestyle and Food Habits, you have a true recipe for lasting health and happiness!

My Favorite Herbs & Oils

Essential Oils

- ∞ Lavender
- ∞ Rosemary
- ∞ Tea Tree
- ∞ Eucalyptus
- ∞ Lemon
- ∞ Peppermint
- ∞ Lemongrass

Herbs

- ∞ Peppermint
- ∞ German Chamomile
- ∞ Rosemary
- ∞ Lavender
- ∞ Garlic
- ∞ Cilantro
- ∞ Turmeric

The quality of essential oils and herbs you choose make a difference in the efficacy of the treatment and results you are seeking. Look for USDA certified organic or wild crafted oils and herbs. You can learn to grow a wide variety of herbs in containers or in your own garden, adding beauty, flavor, and fun to your cooking as well as using them to support your wellbeing. If you choose to purchase instead of grow your own, always purchase your oils and herbs from a trusted resource. Consider asking a health store clerk or qualified aromatherapist for direction. I have my favorite resources for oils and herbs on my website at www.headpositivemom.com, or www.thenourishedlife.net.

There are a variety of different ways to get oils and herbs into your body. For oils, I dilute and apply topically or diffuse. Essential oils are incredibly concentrated and should be treated with respect. *I do not recommend taking oils internally.* Herbs are a little different than oils in that you are presented with the whole plant. Herbal preparations are not typically concentrated (although you can make or purchase concentrated concoctions), and can often be taken internally. Herbs can often show up in our spice cabinet. I cook with herbs, make teas, tinctures, and sometimes mash and make poultices.

Application and use of Herbs and Oils

On the skin: The skin is the largest organ of your body! Your skin acts as a filter, slowly allowing into your body what is applied topically. Once introduced to your body through your skin, your blood delivers the oils and herbs to various organs and body systems.

You may apply essential oils, once diluted with a carrier oil, to almost any area of your body. Avoid sensitive areas like your eyes. Some of the best places to apply an essential oil blend include the bottoms of the feet, inside of your elbows, beneath or behind your ears, and on your chest. After application, be sure to watch for reaction. *If you develop any sort of negative reaction including but not limited to hives, redness, or sensitivity, discontinue use and seek the support of a medical professional.*

Essential oils can be added to your favorite skin care products. Try adding a drop or two to conditioner, body wash, night time face moisturizer, body lotion, or even placing a drop or two in your shoes.

In the bath: Want an incredible, relaxing spa like experience? Next to topical application, taking a warm bath with oils or herbs is an incredibly soothing and effective method of aromatherapy.

Oils - After your tub is filled, add 3 – 15 drops of your favorite essential oil blend. You'll want to wait until you turn the water off to add these oils, then swirl into your bath water using your hands.

Herbs – (Try rose petals or lavender buds) – fill a muslin or tea bag with herbs and leave it in the tub while you bathe. You can do this without the bag, but you'll create quite a mess! Muslin bags and empty tea bags are available at your local vitamin or whole foods stores.

Vaporizing and diffusing: (For essential oils) Purchasing a diffuser made specifically for essential oils is a great idea and allows you to easily introduce these oils into to your environment. The result is a wonderful aromatic space in which you are breathing in the essential oils.

Steam inhalation: This method works for both oils and herbs. You'll need only a pot, towels, and a glass bowl. Boil water and carefully pour boiling water into the glass bowl located where you can lean over it without spilling. Add an oil blend or herbs, then lean your face over the bowl being cautious not to get too close. Cover your head with a towel to trap the steam vapors. Be very careful to not burn yourself with the boiled water, don't touch your face to the water, and don't be afraid to take towel off to breathe if you feel the need. *This application is not recommended for children.*

Sprays: This method works only with oils. Sprays can be easily made for your body or room. To extend the life of your blends, all sprays should be stored in colored glass bottles. For a body spray, blend oils with purified or spring water, rose water, or witch hazel. For a room spray blend oils with purified water. Because oils and water doesn't mix, shake well before every use.

Cleaning products: Replacing chemical cleaners with natural essential oil based homemade cleaners is a great way to minimize toxic exposure in your home. When preparing your own, mix up just enough of the recipe for your immediate use. Essential oils have amazing antiviral and antibacterial properties and leave a lovely scent in your freshly cleaned rooms.

Others: Essential oils can be applied to corners of a room, on cotton balls placed in your drawers, to the corner of a washcloth in your dryer, to the inside of a toilet paper tube (then put on the toilet paper holder), inside your car, and so many other areas! Be creative, start small, and enjoy! You can also make a potpourri using fragrant herbs. These are both decorative and useful.

An Apothecary to Call Your Own

There are mass amounts of options when it comes to setting up your own home apothecary. Just like food, it can serve you plenty to master a few, make a plan, and take it one step at a time. (Remember K.I.S.S.?)

Begin by identifying a few common household ailments and challenges. An example of this might be: stress, anxiety, sleeplessness, colds, allergies, or headaches.

Find a few reliable reference books like Rosemary Gladstar's Family Herbal, or Valerie Ann Worwood's The Complete Book of Essential Oils & Aromatherapy to research common attributes and benefits.

Because herbs are multifaceted, you will find a single herb or oil will support you in a variety of ways. My all around favorite essential oil and herb is Lavender. I always keep a bit of the essential oil around for emergencies of all sorts. I also grow my own so that I can have fresh buds every summer. I am sure with a little research and discovery of your own, you'll find a few of your favorite herbs and essential oils to keep on hand as well.

Oil Blends & Herb recipes to experiment with

Irritating cough?

Steam Inhalation or Diffusing Blend

2 drops lavender
2 drops eucalyptus

Try an herbal tea that includes Peppermint and/ or Licorice root

Head throbbing?

Temple Rub

2 drops lavender and 2 drops peppermint in 1 tsp. carrier oil.

♦   Rub into temples and neck being careful to avoid eyes.

Diffuse

7 drops lavender
3 drops peppermint

Try applying a cool moist washcloth to the base of your skull or over your eyes.

Itchy bug bites?

Apply 1 – 2 drops lavender oil "neat" to area

If it's a bee sting, I will mix a little water and baking soda and apply directly over the area.

Dry and Splitting Hair?

Mix together ¼ cup Coconut oil with 3 – 4 drops rosemary essential oil. Apply to tips of hair and work toward scalp. Leave on for ten minutes and wash with mild shampoo under warm water.

Not sleeping well?

Diffuse or make a spray for sheets and bedroom area

8 drops of lavender
or 8 drops of frankincense

Chamomile tea is especially helpful for calming a person before bed and is generally safe for children as well. My favorite brands are Traditional Medicinals and Celestial Seasonings.

Gotta Burn?

Soak burned area in cool water (or with a cold wet cloth) with 15 drops lavender for about 15 minutes. Lavender may be applied "neat" to the area.

Use the gel of a fresh aloe leaf. I do this by using a knife to split the leaf and scrape the gel from the inside. Apply directly to the burn area. Works great for any type of burn, especially healing post sun exposure.

Snuffly Nose?

Add to Warm Bath Water

2 drops Rosemary
2 drops Eucalyptus
2 drops Lavender

Diffuse

2 drops Lavender
2 drops Tea Tree
2 drops Eucalyptus

Eat raw garlic. No one likes to do this, but garlic is a powerful antiviral, antibacterial herb. To maximize the healing compound, it must be eaten raw and chewed rather than chopped.

Bugs buggin' you?

3 drops Citronella
3 drops Lemongrass
1 tsp. base oil

Blend oils and apply topically to exposed skin areas.

You may also like to make a spray using the above oils and add them to water in lieu of oil. Shake before each use.

Burn Citronella candles

These are just a few of thousands of ideas, blends, and recipes that there are floating around in the world. For more essential oil and herb tips, visit my website at headpositivemom.com or see the resources section for other places I post recipes and ideas.

Part IV – MomPositive Recipes

Cooking for a family can get complicated when you are trying to please everyone, yet still serve healthy and easy to prepare food. When I was at my peak juggling a full time corporate career and the front end of my now thriving Health Coaching practice, I was maxed out time wise. I began to find ways to cut corners and prep time around meals while still empowering my family to make healthy choices.

I found that offering a "serve yourself bar" of any sort allowed my family to choose what appealed most to them, yet I could filter what was offered. We still do a lot of burrito bars, taco bars, and salad bars. I find my family making great choices when they have great foods to choose from.

Use this portion of the workbook to experiment with new foods, learn to cut your own corners, and find fun tasty foods your family will thrive on!

These are just a sampling of recipes available on my website at www.thenourishedlife.net or www.headpositivemom.com.

Coco-Yogurt Parfait
1 cup vanilla coconut yogurt (So Delicious)
¼ cup homemade granola or favorite brand
½ cup mixed berries
½ tsp. flax seed

Layer yogurt, granola and fruit, then sprinkle on whole flax seeds

Serves 1

Peach Smoothie
1 cup original almond milk
1 cup vanilla coconut yogurt
2 cups frozen peaches
8 - 10 raw almonds or walnuts

Add all ingredients to blender, blend until very smooth

Serves 3 -4

Strawberry Bang Smoothie

1 cup coconut milk
1 cup cultured coconut milk (found by the kefir in the refrigerated section)
1 cup frozen strawberries
1 cup chopped spinach
1 tbsp. flax

Place all ingredients in a blender and blend until smooth. Enjoy!

Serves 3 -4

Cran-Apple Smoothie

1 green apple, diced and cored
1 cucumber, peeled and diced
½ cup frozen cranberries
1 cup coconut water
2 cups water

Blend all ingredients until smooth. Serve with a slice of GF multigrain toast and a boiled egg.

Serves 3 – 4

Green Smoothie

2 – 3 leaves romaine lettuce
1/2 cup baby spinach leaves
1 ripe fresh pear (cored)
1 cup frozen blueberries
1 ½ cup original almond milk
1 cup vanilla coconut yogurt
1 tbsp. flax seeds

Blend until smooth. Add more milk or yogurt to make creamier or thinner. Can serve 2 – 3

Happy Tummy Oats

4 cups water, bring to a boil
2 cups steel cut oats
2 granny smith apple, cored and diced
1/2 cup raw walnuts
2 tsp. cinnamon
4 tbsp. maple syrup

Add oats and apples to water and reduce heat to simmer, stir occasionally. Cook for fifteen – twenty minutes. Serve warm, topped with cinnamon, syrup, and walnuts.

Serves 4 – 5

3 Bears Porridge

1 cup leftover quinoa (or leftover brown rice)
½ cup almond milk
¼ cup cranberries or raisins
cinnamon

*optional – maple syrup or honey to sweeten

Place ¼ cup of water in a sauce pan and heat to boiling. Reduce heat, add cold precooked grain, milk and fruit. Heat through, take care to not boil milk, and put into bowls to serve. Top with cinnamon and if you want, sweeten with syrup or honey.

Serves 1 per cup, increase recipe according to number of people eating.

Amazing Eggs and Mushroom Sauté

coconut oil or olive oil
6 eggs
Minced garlic
1tsp turmeric
½ tsp chili powder
1 small zucchini
2 roma tomatoes
6 baby bella mushrooms

Dice all veggies into small bite size pieces. Heat oil in a skillet, over medium heat. Add tomatoes, zucchini, mushrooms, and garlic. Sauté until tender, about three or four minutes. Add turmeric and chili powder. Mix in thoroughly. Remove from pan. (Set aside)

Using the same skillet, make over easy eggs. Using a spatula, shape and unstick eggs from the skillet until yolks are runny but all whites are cooked, turning only once.

Serve with Egg in center of plate, topped with sautéed vegetables. Sprinkle a dash of salt if desired.

May add a whole grain gluten free English muffin or sprouted grain bread to this dish!

Serves 4 – 6

Apple Slices w/ Nut Butter

Use an apple slicer, available at any kitchen goods store. This cuts the apple into even, easy to eat slices. Dip into your favorite nut butter. For weight loss, limit your nut butter to 2 tablespoons.

Strawberry Avocado Salad

4 tbsp extra virgin olive oil
10 tsp raw honey
2 tbsp cider vinegar
2 tsp lemon juice
4 cups mixed salad greens
2 avocados - peeled, pitted and sliced
20 strawberries, sliced
1 cup chopped walnuts

In a small bowl, mix together olive oil, honey, vinegar, and lemon juice. Set aside.
Rinse salad greens, and spin dry in a salad spinner. Put greens in a medium bowl. Top with avocado and strawberry slices. Serve vinaigrette on the side for each person to top as they wish. Top with a sprinkling of walnuts

Serves 4

Simple Vinaigrette

¼ cup extra virgin olive oil
4 tsp red wine vinegar
½ tsp sea salt
freshly ground pepper to taste

Serve over any fresh green salad.

Rainbow of Flavor Sauté

In your favorite skillet, add 2 tbsp. Olive Oil and heat over medium heat. Add all below chopped vegetables:
zucchini
yellow squash
red sweet pepper
celery
black pepper
2 cloves minced garlic
1 tsp. turmeric

Sauté until vegetables begin to soften. Add to soups, stews, top rice or quinoa, or put in a gluten free wrap. Simple and tasty!

Veggie Taco Chili

1 can organic black beans
1 can organic pinto beans
1 large can Muir Glen Roasted Tomatoes (Diced)
1 can mild green chilies
1 tsp. canned or fresh jalapenos
2 cups vegetable broth
1 cup water
1 tbsp. cumin
1 tbsp. paprika
1 tsp. sea salt
2 tsp. pepper
1 clove fresh minced garlic
2 stalks (about ¼ cup chopped) fresh parsley

In a large pot add all ingredients and cook until heated through, about 20 to 25 minutes, stirring frequently.

Easily Serves 4, served with flax crackers

Sweet Potato Soft Tacos

1 package GF taco size wraps or tortillas, I like to use the Rudi's brand
3 small or 2 medium sweet potatoes, peeled & cut into fries, baked at 375° F. until soft
3 tbsp. olive oil
½ head chopped romaine lettuce
2 chopped roma tomatoes
sweet peppers
¾ cup fresh chopped cilantro
black olives
1 avocado, smash thoroughly
Your favorite salsa

Create a taco bar by offering all your ingredients separately. Allow each person to build his/her own taco.

Pizza Night

Gluten Free Pizza Crust (I use Bob's Red Mill)
fresh tomato
fresh basil
olive oil
pesto
minced garlic
green or black olives
spinach
*optional dairy free cheese, we just like to eat it without

Bake Crust according to package directions. Layer tomato, basil, spinach, olives, pesto (contains dairy), etc.; as you desire. Toast in oven until all toppings are warmed through at 375°F for about ten minutes. Edges will have turned lightly brown. I love using olive oil in place of tomato sauce.

Broccoli Salad

¼ cup balsamic vinegar
2 tbsp. dijon mustard
2 tbsp. honey
¼ tsp. Himalayan sea salt
¼ pepper
4 tbsp. olive oil
2 heads broccoli
1 small red onion
½ cup whole almonds, raw
½ cup dried cranberries

In a large bowl mix together vinegar, mustard, honey, salt and pepper. Whisk in oil until well blended. Set aside.

Remove broccoli florets from stalk and add to vinaigrette. Add onion, almonds, and cranberries to the bowl. Toss and serve.

Tri-Color Peppers & Steak

1 Pkg. Frozen Peppers – Tricolored
2 Beef Filets
¼ White Onion
2 cloves garlic minced
Olive Oil
Sea Salt

Remove steaks from fridge and set out in plastic or glass container. Drizzle with olive oil and top with sea salt. Allow to come to room temperature. Heat skillet over medium heat. Sauté garlic, onion and peppers until just before soft. Remove from pan and set aside. While peppers are cooking, slice steak into thin strips, against the grain. Cook in same skillet as peppers, until cooked through – about 5 -10 minutes. Serve over peppers. May opt to serve with rice or quinoa.

Burritos

GF Tortillas
1 Can Organic vegetarian pinto beans, rinse & drain
¼ Yellow onion, diced
1 ripe avocado

1 sweet red pepper
2 cups chopped mixed greens
Favorite Salsa

Lay 1 tortilla flat on each plate and layer ingredients as desired.

Super Easy Grilled Chicken & Veggies
(Chicken Foil Pack)

1 pound organic free range skinless, boneless chicken breast – cubed**
2 onions, diced
1 (8 ounce) package sliced fresh mushrooms
1 green bell pepper, seeded and sliced into strips
1 red bell pepper, seeded and sliced into strips
4 cloves of garlic, sliced or minced
4 small potatoes, cubed
1/4 cup extra virgin olive oil
1 lemon
1 roll aluminum foil, tear off four large (10 – 12")

Preheat grill to high.
Lay foil flat. In a large bowl, combine all ingredients. Using a large spoon or ladle, put a big scoop (or two) onto each sheet of foil. Fold foil around food to fully enclose. Seal edges tightly.
Reduce grill heat to medium. Place foil packs on grill for about 30 minutes, chicken needs to be fully done and potatoes tender.
Serve warm.

Serves 4.
** Easily turn this into a vegetarian dish by eliminating chicken.

These are just a sampling of recipes available on my website at www.thenourishedlife.net or www.headpositivemom.com.

Putting It All Together

If you are reading this, you've either made it through the entire workbook, or you've cut straight to the back. I almost always read my health books this way. Back first. If that's the case, you'll be happy to know that this journey is not about achieving perfection. It's about finding what works for Y-O-U in your life, in *your* body.

One step at a time, one idea and one new habit at a time. If you find you are ready to move on, trust yourself and move on! If you haven't quite mastered a topic but feel like it would be really helpful for you....trust yourself, stick with that topic until you master it!

Not every day will be perfect, and that's okay. What will make the greatest difference is taking each day as it comes, learning to be flexible, creative, and patient – *with you*.

Each new day is a chance to start fresh. Even after those days you feel like you've totally bailed on yourself and binged on everything in sight, you are able to take a deep breath, let it go, and look ahead to your next choice.

By simply asking yourself, "what will I do differently next time? ", opens the doorway to that next step.

Every day you choose *you, your* wellbeing, *your* happiness and healthiness, you are able to show up more for those you love beyond measure.

The magic sauce is action. You get out of it, what you put into it.

So, if you are reading this first, there's no magic formula here, except go back to the front of the book and begin. If you are finishing this workbook with this note, then you should **CELEBRATE** your new, reinvented **Y-O-U**!

YOU DID IT MOMMA!

About the Author

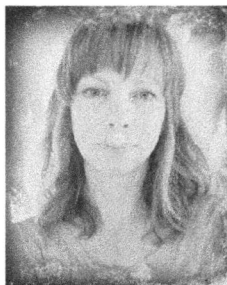

Since 2004, Tammi has been on a quest to discover, live, and share the life and health benefits of natural living. She is a Board Certified Integrative Nutrition Health Coach, Aromatherapist, and Herbalist, with a passion for helping busy professional and entrepreneurial Moms lead balanced, abundant, and healthy lives.

Tammi teaches from both personal life experience and an abundance of natural health education that includes graduating from the world's largest nutrition school, The Institute for Integrative Nutrition. It was at The Institute for Integrative Nutrition that she studied with the world's top health and nutrition experts including: Joshua Rosenthal, David Wolfe, Joel Fuhrman, Dr. David Katz, Dr. Andrew Weil, Gabrielle Bernstein, and Geneen Roth.

In July 2012, Tammi was awarded the Health Leadership Award, by The Institute for Integrative Nutrition.

She has also earned certification and training as follows:

2005 - American College of Health Sciences - Master Herbalist Diploma
2010 - Institute for Integrative Nutrition - Health Coach Professional Training Program
2011 - Institute for Integrative Nutrition - Immersion Studies
2012 - Penn Foster - Holistic Nutrition
2012 - The University of Arizona - Environmental Medicine – An Integrative Approach
2013 - UCSF - (Coursera) - Nutrition for Health Promotion and Disease Prevention
2013 - Integrated Healing Solutions – Usui Reiki I & II
2014 - Holistic Arts Institute - Aromatherapy Essentials
2014 - Holistic Arts Institute - Aromatherapy Healing Arts
2014 - American Fitness Professionals Associates - Nutrition & Wellness Coach
2014 - American Fitness Professionals Associates - Sports Nutrition

Tammi has been professionally certified with the American Association of Drugless Practitioners and is a proud Member of IAHC, The International Association of Health Coaches.

Aside from her passions in natural health, Tammi is happily married to the love of her life, the incredibly proud mother of two, and grandmother of one. Her hobbies include gardening, scrapbooking, soap making, cooking, reading nutrition and health books, caring for her furr babies, and exploring this great world.

MomPositive Health Coaching Resources

To contact Tammi please email or use a contact form from one of her websites below.

Want more? Tammi wants to share more with you! Be sure you stop by her website to down load free guides, get free recipes, schedule a free fifty minute consultation, and learn more about living MomPositively!

www.headpositivemom.com OR www.thenourishedlife.net

I am here to help you succeed!

Tammi Hoerner, INHC

tammihoerner@gmail.com

www.headpositivemom.com

www.thenourishedlife.net

Follow Tammi on Facebook at: https://www.facebook.com/tammi.hoerner

Follow Tammi on Pinterest at: https://www.pinterest.com/tammihoerner/

Additional Resources:

The Institute for Integrative Nutrition

Learn more about being an Integrative Nutrition Health Coach here: http://geti.in/1wfnjHA

Resources & References

1. "Hydrate." The Free Dictionary by Farlex. http://www.thefreedictionary.com/hydrating. 18. June 2015

2. Knapp, Julie. "15 houseplants for improving indoor air quality." Mother Nature Network. MNN Holding Company, LLC. http://www.mnn.com/health/healthy-spaces/photos/15-houseplants-for-improving-indoor-air-quality/a-breath-of-fresh-air. 21. June. 2015.

3. Magee, Elaine MPH RD., and Chang, Louise MD. "Can a Food Diary Help You Lose Weight?"WebMD. MedicineNet.com. 26. September. 2008. http://www.webmd.com/diet/obesity/can-food-diary-help-you-lose-weight. 16. June. 2015.

4. "Migraine Fact Sheet." Migraine Research Foundation. http://www.migraineresearchfoundation.org/fact-sheet.html. 19. June. 2015
In text citation, page 18.

5. Weil, Andrew MD. Spontaneous Happiness. Weil. Little Brown and Company. 8. November. 2011. "Generalized Anxiety Disorder." http://www.drweil.com/drw/u/ART00695/generalized-anxiety-disorder.html. 17. June. 2015

    4.   The Institute for Integrative Nutrition and IIN are trademarks of Integrative Nutrition Inc.

Journal & Schedule

Morning thoughts:
_____
_____
_____
_____
_____
_____
_____

Goals & Intentions for today

1
2
3
4
5
6

6:00	
7:00	
8:00	
9:00	
10:00	
11:00	
12:00	
1:00	
2:00	
3:00	
4:00	
5:00	
6:00	
7:00	

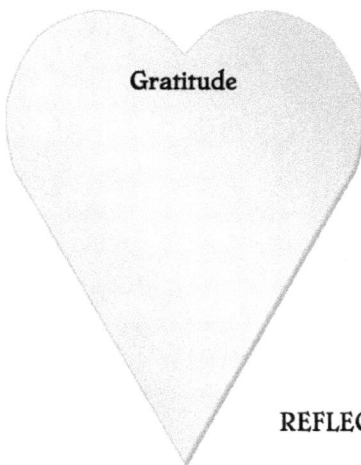

Food

Water: IIII IIII IIII

Breakfast:
_____
_____
_____

Lunch:
_____
_____
_____

Dinner:
_____
_____
_____

Snacks:
_____
_____

Notes:
_____
_____
_____

Gratitude

REFLECTION
_____
_____
_____
_____
_____
_____

www.ingramcontent.com/pod-product-compliance
Lightning Source LLC
Chambersburg PA
CBHW08047280326
41934CB00014B/3238